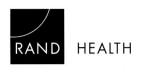

RAND HEALTH

T0262422

Toward a Sustainable Blood Supply in the United States

An Analysis of the Current System and Alternatives for the Future

Andrew W. Mulcahy, Kandice A. Kapinos, Brian Briscombe,
Lori Uscher-Pines, Ritika Chaturvedi, Spencer R. Case,
Jakub Hlávka, Benjamin M. Miller

Sponsored by the U.S. Department of Health and Human Services

For more information on this publication, visit www.rand.org/t/RR1575

Library of Congress Cataloging-in-Publication Data is available for this publication

ISBN: 978-0-8330-9679-1

Published by the RAND Corporation, Santa Monica, Calif.
© Copyright 2016 RAND Corporation
RAND® is a registered trademark.

Cover images: stockerteam / iStock / Getty Images;
Jochen Sands / DigitalVision / Getty Images

Support RAND
Make a tax-deductible charitable contribution at
www.rand.org/giving/contribute

www.rand.org

Preface

A robust, sustainable blood system is a crucial component of every health care system. The availability of safe blood and blood products is a prerequisite for various health care services—including some surgeries, treatments for cancer and other acute and chronic medical conditions, trauma care, organ transplantation, and childbirths—that extend and improve life for millions of patients annually.

This report describes the status quo in the U.S. blood system, explores a set of research questions related to the sustainability of the U.S. blood system through analysis and discussion, and presents policy alternatives and tools to help ensure that the U.S. blood system is sustainable. We employed a mixed-methods approach, blending insight from analyses of available data and from a series of interviews and other interactions with stakeholder groups. The report is targeted to federal policymakers with a role in the regulation and functioning of the blood supply, payment for services involving blood, and public investment in innovation.

This research was sponsored by the U.S. Department of Health and Human Services (HHS), Office of the Assistant Secretary of Health (OASH), and conducted by RAND Health, a division of the RAND Corporation. A profile of RAND Health, abstracts of its publications, and ordering information can be found at www.rand.org/health.

This research was conducted under contract HHSP233201500038I/HHSP23337002T with HHS. The Project Officer for the project was Rich Henry of HHS, OASH. We thank him for his guidance and review of the document; however, we note that the material contained in this report is the responsibility of the research team and does not necessarily reflect the beliefs or opinions of HHS, OASH, or the federal government.

Contents

Figures

Tables

Summary

A robust, sustainable blood system is a crucial component of every health care system. The availability of safe blood and blood products is a prerequisite for various health care services—including some surgeries, treatments for cancer and other acute and chronic medical conditions, trauma care, organ transplantation, and childbirths—that extend and improve life for millions of patients annually.

The current U.S. blood system is built from the coordinated activities of multiple stakeholder groups. Volunteer donors supply almost all blood and its components, which are tested, processed, stocked, and distributed by nonprofit blood centers. Blood centers supply hospitals and other health care providers that use blood or keep blood on hand to deliver health care services to patients. These hospitals—rather than blood centers—are then paid for the health care services by Medicare and other public and private health care payers. In most cases, the same payment is made to hospitals regardless of whether blood was used. More broadly, the U.S. Food and Drug Administration (FDA) regulates the collection, processing, testing, and other aspects of the blood system. The Centers for Disease Control and Prevention (CDC) works together with the U.S. Biovigilance Network to monitor the U.S. blood system. The National Institutes of Health supports and conducts research to improve collection, transfusion, and management of the nation's blood resources.

Several factors are placing stress on the U.S. blood system—and, in particular, on blood centers and their suppliers. First, while the functioning of the blood system in terms of centers' capacity to collect and supply blood has remained relatively constant over time, the demand for blood has decreased markedly in the past decade, mainly because of changes in clinical practice. The result has been a downward shift in the market price that hospitals pay blood centers for blood, thereby reducing blood center margins and revenue. Second, ongoing consolidation among hospitals has added to the financial stress on blood centers and suppliers of blood-related equipment, goods, and services by shifting negotiating power toward buyers. Third, technological innovation and the emergence of new pathogens, such as the Zika virus, add new costs to the production and testing of blood. Blood centers report that it is difficult to pass on these additional production and testing costs to buyers. Taken together, these stresses are pressuring the U.S. blood system to evolve, possibly toward a more-sustainable system in the long term, but potentially with some short-term negative consequences through the transition.

We define a *sustainable blood system* as one that (1) maintains or improves on current safety levels for blood and blood products, (2) provides blood for the full range of clinical applications consistent with standard practice, and (3) delivers blood in a timely fashion such that patient health and preparedness are not unduly compromised. A system will be more likely to meet these criteria if it maintains incentives for innovation, operates efficiently in terms of production and delivery, minimizes disruptions from routine market changes, and has sufficient surge capacity to cope with emergencies and other significant disruptions.

This report describes the status quo in the U.S. blood system, explores a set of six specific research questions related to the sustainability of the U.S. blood system through analysis and discussion, and presents policy alternatives and tools to help ensure that the U.S. blood system is sustainable. We employed a mixed-methods approach, blending insight from analyses of available data and from a series of interviews and other interactions with stakeholder groups. The six specific research questions we addressed are:

1. How do blood system stakeholders perceive the main trends in the U.S. health care system, and how do these trends influence the current and future sustainability of the U.S. blood system?
2. How could changes in payment for health care services and blood affect the sustainability of the U.S. blood system?
3. What is the insurance value of blood—that is, the value that hospitals, patients, and society derive from having a safe blood supply readily accessible in the event of an emergency? To what extent does the price that hospitals and society pay capture this value?
4. What are the key potential public health risks to sustainability from emergencies?
5. What are the potential effects of new business models, including brokerage models?
6. What best practices do we observe in other nations' blood systems that can be practically applied to improve the U.S. blood system?

We stress an important distinction between ensuring a sustainable blood system and sustaining the status quo in the blood system. Our analyses and recommendations recognize that the path toward a more-sustainable blood system might involve significant changes in the structure of the blood industry, financial arrangements between different stakeholders, and the role of the government in the blood system. At the same time, unexpected and sudden departures from the status quo—for example, the closure of blood centers for financial reasons—might result in undesirable consequences in the short term without policy intervention, even if these changes promote the long-term sustainability of the system.

This report includes a brief introduction (Chapter One), a description of the U.S. blood system (Chapter Two), a summary of our study methods (Chapter Three), separate chapters addressing each of the six research questions (Chapters Four through Nine), and a final chapter (Chapter Ten) describing shared themes and recommendations to the U.S. Department of Health and Human Services (HHS).

Findings

The main findings related to the six research questions are as follows (in order, by chapter):

Leading trends affecting the blood sector include reduced demand for blood, shrinking profits for blood centers and their suppliers, a shrinking pool of active donors, hospital consolidation, and blood center alliances or consolidation.

A set of alternative payment policies could mitigate short-term pressures on the blood system (if, in fact, this is the policy goal), but it is important to consider the status quo as an important policy option, particularly given its advantages in terms of incentives for price competition.

Available blood that is not being immediately used has value to society, hospitals, and patients. There is risk or uncertainty that individual hospitals might not have enough blood in the event of an emergency, and there is also society-level risk that an event could occur that would threaten the blood system's ability to meet demand in an emergency. Alternative market mechanisms could mitigate these risks.

The key emergency public health risks to sustainability include natural disasters, terrorist attacks, and pandemics. Each varies in its potential effects on the blood system, including unknown onset, likely impacts, and consequences on supply and demand. Defining and then maintaining appropriate levels of surge capacity will help to address these various types of emergency risk.

Business models shaping the landscape of blood provision include nationally integrated organizations, local independent organizations, and blood brokerages. Various trends affect each model differently, and the expansion of each model carries different implications to the blood system.

Best practices observed in selected foreign countries include effective hemovigilance (HV) programs, improved regulatory environment for medical devices, and more-coordinated government support for research and development (R&D). Strengthening U.S. HV would require increasing participation in the U.S. HV reporting systems; improving data accuracy by increasing adherence to HV case definitions; and centralizing HV data aggregation, analysis, and results dissemination. Policymakers could also improve the regulatory environment for medical devices by increasing the speed and decreasing the cost of regulatory approvals for such devices and by harmonizing with or converging toward internationally prevalent blood safety standards. U.S. policymakers could further encourage investments in R&D by sustaining or expanding government blood-related R&D investments and more closely coordinating the investments of blood centers, suppliers, and government funders.

Recommendations

Based on these findings, we make the following recommendations to improve the sustainability of the U.S. blood system:

Collect data on blood use and financial arrangements. While stakeholders have access to statistics on blood use and transactions related to their individual organizations, the U.S. government currently does not have access to comprehensive data describing the performance of the blood system as a whole.

Develop and disseminate a vision for appropriate levels of surge capacity. Describing a desired level of surge capacity from a public health and preparedness perspective will help stakeholders and policymakers plan and estimate the costs associated with maintaining surge capacity in the blood system aside from the usual transaction-based arrangements between blood centers and hospitals.

Subsidize blood centers' ability to maintain surge capacity. Surge capacity to respond to serious events and emergencies falls outside the typical financial arrangements between hospitals and blood centers. During the current environment of falling demand for blood and resulting excess supply, centers have shown some surge capacity to meet emergency needs. However, once the industry has adjusted to lower demand, there is no guarantee that this surge capacity will remain. If blood centers are asked to retain excess staff, collection capabilities, or stock for any reason other than meeting the current demand for blood from hospitals, there is a strong argument that the government should separately finance this surge capacity.

Build relationships with brokers and other entities to form a blood "safety net." HHS should build ongoing relationships with the American Red Cross, the Armed Services Blood Program, and brokerage entities that would commit to procuring and delivering blood at the request of HHS to address short-term and local shortages. A well-established set of relationships can reduce response times in the case of shortages.

Build and implement a value framework for new technology. We recommend that HHS invest in health technology assessment research for existing technologies with low adoption rates and for technologies on the horizon. These analyses should distinguish between costs and benefits accruing to blood centers and hospitals and costs and benefits from the broader societal perspective. For technologies with significant costs and benefits from the societal perspective but not from the blood center and hospital perspectives, policy intervention could encourage adoption.

Pay directly for new technologies for which there is no private business case for adoption. Decisions to adopt some tests that are now industry standards are difficult to justify from the business perspectives of blood centers and hospitals. However, these technologies often have clear public health and preparedness benefits, so policymakers might want to require or at least encourage adoption. In these cases, U.S. government financing of technology acquisition costs might be appropriate.

Implement emergency use authorization and contingency planning for key supplies and inputs. HHS could—through FDA—implement emergency use authorizations for replacement supplies and other inputs in the event of a shortage.

Acknowledgments

We would like to thank several staff at the U.S. Department of Health and Human Services (HHS), Office of the Assistant Secretary of Health (OASH), including Rich Henry and Jim Berger for their support and guidance. We also appreciate the helpful comments on earlier drafts of this report from members of the HHS Blood, Organ, and Tissue Senior Executive Council.

We want to express our gratitude to all members of the Advisory Committee on Blood and Tissue Safety and Availability, an advisory committee that provides guidance to the federal government on a range of policy issues related to blood, blood products, and tissues, for helping us refine our research questions and providing expertise when needed. We are especially thankful to members who helped facilitate discussions with other key stakeholders. We thank all of the blood centers, hospitals, blood system suppliers, and providers who were willing to talk to us repeatedly in providing invaluable insight and data to our analysis. We thank Alan Williams at the Food and Drug Administration for providing us with the publicly available blood establishment registry data. We also greatly appreciate informative conversations with the following experts in the field: W. Keith Hoots and Harvey Klein at the National Institutes of Health, Jacqueline Little at the Food and Drug Administration, Gary Disbrow in the Office of the Assistant Secretary for Preparedness and Response, and blood bank expert Michael Strong. In addition to those contributors, we thank a number of other individuals and organizations that participated anonymously.

Abbreviations

AABB	formerly known as the American Association of Blood Banks
ABC	America's Blood Centers
ACA	Affordable Care Act
ACO	accountable care organization
AOR	After Outliers Removed
APC	ambulatory payment classification
ASPR	Office of the Assistant Secretary for Preparedness and Response
ARC	American Red Cross
ARCBS	Australian Red Cross Blood Service
ASBP	Armed Services Blood Program
BARDA	Biomedical Advanced Research and Development Authority
BASIS	Blood Availability and Safety Information System
BCA	Blood Centers of America
BLA	Biologics License Application
BOR	Before Outliers Removed
BSI	Blood Systems Inc.
CBER	Center for Biologics Evaluation and Research
CBS	Canadian Blood Services
CDC	Centers for Disease Control and Prevention
CMS	Centers for Medicare & Medicaid Services
CPS	Center for Patient Safety

CPT	Current Procedural Terminology
CRC	Canadian Red Cross
DBSH	Disproportionate Blood Share Hospital
DoD	U.S. Department of Defense
DRG	diagnosis-related group
DSH	Disproportionate Share Hospital
EIM	Electronic Inventory Management
EU	European Union
FDA	U.S. Food and Drug Administration
FQHC	federally qualified health centers
FTE	full-time equivalent
FY	fiscal year
GAO	U.S. General Accountability Office
GMP	Good Manufacturing Practices
GPO	group purchasing organization
HBV	hepatitis B virus
HCPCS	Healthcare Common Procedure Coding System
HCV	hepatitis C virus
HHI	Herfindahl-Hirschman Index
HHS	U.S. Department of Health and Human Services
HIV	human immunodeficiency virus
HOPD	hospital outpatient department
HRR	hospital referral region
HRSA	Health Resources and Services Administration
HV	hemovigilance
ICU	intensive care unit
IOPO	independent organ procurement organization
IPPS	Inpatient Prospective Payment System
IT	information technology

JRCS	Japan Red Cross Society
MAA	marketing authorization application
MDET	medical device excise tax
ML	medical license
MS-DRG	Medicare severity-adjusted diagnosis-related group
NBA	National Blood Authority
NBCUS	National Blood Collection and Utilization Survey
NBE	National Blood Exchange
NHSBT	National Health Service Blood and Transplant
NHSN	National Healthcare Safety Network
NIH	National Institutes of Health
NTAP	new technology add-on payment
OASH	Office of the Assistant Secretary of Health
OPPS	outpatient prospective payment system
PEI	Paul-Ehrlich-Institut
PESTL	political, economic, sociocultural, technological, and legal
PFS	Physician Fee Schedule
PHAC	Public Health Agency of Canada
PR	pathogen reduction
PRT	pathogen reduction technology
RBC	red blood cell
R&D	research and development
RFP	request for proposal
SHOT	Serious Hazards of Transfusion
SOC	U.S. Department of Health and Human Services Secretary's Office of Operations
SNF	skilled nursing facility
TACO	transfusion-associated circulatory overload
TRALI	transfusion-related acute lung injury

TTISS	Transfusion Transmitted Injuries Surveillance System
UK	United Kingdom
VA	U.S. Department of Veterans Affairs
VHA	Veterans Health Administration
WBA	whole blood automation
WHO	World Health Organization

CHAPTER ONE

Introduction

Blood and blood products (such as plasma and platelets, hereafter referred to collectively as *blood*) are critical inputs into a wide range of medical procedures and services, including surgeries, trauma care, and therapeutic interventions. The U.S. blood system collects, tests, processes, and distributes the blood ultimately used in clinical practice. In 2013, approximately 14.2 million units of blood were collected in the United States from approximately 15.2 million individuals presenting to donate, 13.2 million units of which were transfused.[1] Blood is an input into approximately 10 percent to 15 percent of hospital inpatient stays.[2] The history of blood transfusions as lifesaving procedures is well documented in the literature with estimates that tens of millions of lives have been saved from transfusions.[3]

The U.S. blood system is complex. Blood centers—nonprofit entities, such as the American Red Cross (ARC), that may have multiple physical locations—rely on altruistic blood donors and for-profit equipment and testing suppliers for critical inputs. Nearly 81 percent of plasma donors are compensated in the United States.[4] However, the cost to process plasma is significantly lower than the cost of whole blood, and plasma can be frozen easily thus extending its shelf life substantially. Although previous literature has discussed the possibility of a paid donor pool for whole blood,[5] there

---

[1] K. W. Chung, S. V. Basavaraju, Y. Mu, K. L. van Santen, K. A. Haass, R. Henry, J. Berger, and M. J. Kuehnert, "Declining Blood Collection and Utilization in the United States," *Transfusion*, Vol. 56, Issue 9, May 12, 2016, pp. 2184–2192. Chung et al. report 95-percent confidence intervals of 13.6 million to 14.8 million units collected, 14.4 million to 16.0 million individuals presenting to donate, and 12.4 million to 14.0 million units transfused.

[2] C. Allison Russo and Anne Elixhauser, "Hospitalizations in the Elderly Population, 2003," Statistical Brief No. 6, Agency for Healthcare Research and Quality, May 2006; Anne Pfuntner, Lauren Wier, and Carol Stocks, "Most Frequent Procedures Performed in U.S. Hospitals, 2011," Statistical Brief No. 165, Agency for Healthcare Research and Quality, October 2013.

[3] Robert Slonim, Carmen Wang, and Ellen Garbarino, "The Market for Blood," *The Journal of Economic Perspectives*, Vol. 28, No. 2, 2014, pp. 177–196.

[4] Philip Flood, Peter Wills, Peter Lawler, Graeme Ryan, and Kevin A. Rickard, "Review of Australia's Plasma Fractionation Arrangements," Australian Government Department of Health, 2006.

[5] Slonim, Wang, and Garbarino, 2014.

is considerable controversy surrounding these proposals. As a result, we primarily considered the market for whole blood with volunteer donors (and not plasma) for this report.

Despite these unique characteristics of blood as a product, it is intrinsically a commodity input into the provision of health care, and there exists a competitive market for blood, nonprofit blood centers enter into supply agreements with hospitals, often competing with one another for hospital and regional market share. The most common supply agreement between blood centers and hospitals is a consignment arrangement in which blood centers deliver blood to hospitals, where it is stored, but blood centers are only paid by the hospitals if and when the blood is used. Regulators, blood centers, hospitals, and clinicians strive to maintain the overall safety of the blood supply by providing guidelines and regulations. All of these parties operate in a fragmented and rapidly evolving broader health care system.

Several factors are placing stress on some blood system stakeholders and, in particular, blood centers. Most importantly, the demand for blood is declining because of an increase in patient blood management programs, less-invasive surgeries, pharmacologic agents that eliminate the need for blood transfusions in some situations, and revised transfusion guidelines from professional societies (e.g., lower hemoglobin and platelet count thresholds) that reduce the number of patient transfusions.[6] These developments have increased patient safety while decreasing blood center revenues.

Relatedly, blood center per-unit margins have shrunk. Competition between blood centers—facilitated in some cases by new blood business models, hospital consolidation, and an increasing focus on the part of hospitals to control costs—have contributed to lower prices for blood, while collection, processing, and testing costs either are stable or have increased. As a result, blood centers in particular are facing financial stress. This stress has the potential to affect other stakeholder groups in the blood system—for example, suppliers of equipment, goods, and services to blood centers—and could also reduce blood center investments in research, innovation, and surge capacity. Despite these financial pressures, the blood system has continued to function effectively. However, in the midterm to long term, there are concerns that continued stress on blood centers could eventually affect the timely availability of safe blood products.

The health care market has also changed significantly in recent years and continues to evolve in response to the passage of the Affordable Care Act (ACA), which

---

[6]   Steve Negin, "The Changing Landscape of Blood Banking," *Advance Healthcare Network*, Vol. 24, No. 4, March 26, 2015, p. 28; P. Marks, J. S. Epstein, and L. Borio, "Maintaining a Safe Blood Supply in an Era of Emerging Pathogens," *Journal of Infectious Diseases*, March 8, 2016; A. E. Nielsen and N. D. Nielsen, Assessing Productive Efficiency and Operating Scale of Community Blood Centers," *Transfusion*, February 1, 2016; J. McCullough, J. M. McCullough, and W. J. Riley, "Evolution of the Nation's Blood Supply System," *Transfusion*, April 4, 2016.

has resulted in nearly 20 million newly insured Americans.[7] The provider market is consolidating vertically and horizontally. Nearly 62 percent of community hospitals surveyed by the American Hospital Association are now part of a larger health system (up from about 50 percent in 1999).[8] In addition, a growing number of accountable care organizations (ACOs) and other organizations and programs aim to better integrate care to achieve cost savings and improve quality of care. These changes in market structure, together with more-nimble logistic networks, have significant implications for the bargaining power of hospitals in negotiating arrangements with blood centers. These same changes also create stronger demand for larger blood centers with the scale to supply growing health care delivery systems, while creating new challenges for smaller, regional blood centers.

The ACA also furthered changes to the Centers for Medicare & Medicaid Services' (CMS's) approach to paying for health care services, with greater movement toward bundling payment for episodes of care to incentivize appropriate use of care and cost control. Even prior to the ACA, public and private insurers were experimenting with these innovative payment models, implementing, for example, shared savings arrangements in which payers and providers both benefit if total patient costs are reduced. The growing interest in these payment models—coupled with increasing centralization of purchasing decisions in large hospital chains—can drive hospitals and payers to inspect prices closely for inputs used in the health care system, including blood, some prescription drugs, medical devices, and labor.

The broader regulatory landscape is also changing in ways that affect the blood system. The U.S. Food and Drug Administration (FDA), which is responsible for regulating biological and related products, including blood and blood components, recently amended donor eligibility and testing requirements to improve FDA's ability to respond to new and emerging infectious agents (effective May 2016).[9] FDA rules affect production costs and safety throughout the blood system and will continue to evolve as new pathogens and other challenges emerge.

---

[7] Office of the Assistant Secretary for Planning and Evaluation, "Health Insurance Coverage and the Affordable Care Act," ASPE Data Point, September 22, 2015.

[8] David. M. Cutler and Fiona Scott Morton, "Hospitals, Market Share, and Consolidation," *JAMA*, Vol. 310, No. 18, 2013, pp. 1964–1970.

[9] FDA, "Requirements for Blood and Blood Components Intended for Transfusion or for Further Manufacturing Use," *Federal Register*, Vol. 80, No. 99, May 22, 2015.

The confluence of the decline in demand for blood overall; type-specific, seasonal, or specialized product shortages[10,11]; supply disruptions caused by product recalls and pathogens like the Zika virus; regulatory amendments that increase testing costs; and broader health care market changes raise concerns about the sustainability of the current U.S. blood system. Complicating the difficulty of identifying solutions is the fact that little empirical research has been conducted on the challenges facing the blood system or the likely effects of potential changes to the system. For example, we know little about whether patients systematically have adequate access to blood products, whether incidences of transfusion-related adverse events are rising or falling, whether procedures are being canceled or delayed because of blood availability, and whether there is sufficient surge capacity in the system to respond to large-scale emergencies.

This report aims to identify or fill some of these knowledge gaps, offer objective insights regarding the sustainability of the U.S. blood system, and suggest policy changes that could improve the sustainability of the U.S. blood system. Specifically, this report has the following three primary objectives:

- Describe the current blood system, with a focus on relationships among key players and areas where market inefficiencies might exist.
- Outline potential opportunities to improve any identified inefficiencies and challenges under the current system and explore the potential effects from changes in health care delivery, payment, technology, and clinical practice on blood supply, safety, and prices.
- Propose actionable solutions to the problems identified.

This analysis is grounded in multidisciplinary theories in economics, health policy, and operations management. We use a mixed-methods approach that combines insights from empirical analyses of available data with qualitative inputs from interviews and other interactions with key stakeholder groups.

In Chapter Two, we describe the U.S. blood system status quo, including key stakeholders and steps in the vein-to-vein process run by the blood system, and discuss key stresses on the system. This chapter is intended to serve as a primer for those unfamiliar with the structure of the U.S. blood system and set the stage for later chapters in which we aim to answer more specific questions about how the system is changing and how policies might affect these changes.

---

[10] Stephen Nightingale, Virginia Wanamaker, Barbara Silverman, Paul McCurdy, Lawrence McMurtry, Philip Quarles, S. Gerald Sandler, Darrell Triulzi, Carolyn Whitsett, Christopher Hillyer, Leo McCarthy, Dennis Goldfinger, and David Satcher, "Use of Sentinel Sites for Daily Monitoring of the U.S. Blood Supply," *Transfusion*, Vol. 43, No. 3, 2003, pp. 364–372.

[11] U.S. General Accounting Office (GAO), "Blood Supply Generally Adequate Despite New Donor Restrictions," GAO-02-754, Washington, D.C., July 22, 2002.

The remainder of the report is organized in chapters that align with specific research questions related to the sustainability of the U.S. blood system:

- How do trends in the broader U.S. health care system affect the sustainability of the U.S. blood system?
- How could changes in payment for health care services and blood affect the sustainability of the U.S. blood system?
- What is the insurance value of blood, and can this value be estimated empirically?
- What are the risks to sustainability from emergencies?
- What are the potential impacts of new business models, including brokerage models?
- What best practices do we observe in other nations' blood systems that can be practically applied to improve the U.S. blood system?

These six specific questions were selected from a list of research questions developed by the U.S. Department of Health and Human Services (HHS), Office of the Assistant Secretary of Health (OASH), with refinements and additional research questions suggested by RAND researchers.

Chapter Ten synthesizes findings from the entire report, describes a set of policy alternatives with the potential to strengthen the sustainability of the U.S. blood system, and analyzes the likely impacts of each alternative. In that chapter, we close with recommendations to HHS.

CHAPTER TWO

Overview of the U.S. Blood System

In this chapter, we provide a brief overview of the U.S. blood system, including key stakeholders, steps from donation to use (a vein-to-vein process), and the regulatory and policy context. This chapter is intended for readers who may not already be familiar with all aspects of the U.S. blood system.

Stakeholders

The U.S. blood system involves a range of actors, including donors; blood centers; suppliers of equipment, goods, and services used in the blood system; hospitals and clinicians; and patients. There are also important stakeholders—for example, the Armed Services Blood Program (ASBP), which supports the military and their beneficiaries— that operate separately or in concert with the broader blood system, depending on context and circumstance. In Figure 2.1, we show the distribution of blood establishments in the United States registered with FDA; this does not represent all stakeholders and might not be exhaustive, but it provides an overview of the types and breadth of activity of regulated blood system establishments in the United States. Establishments required to register with FDA include not only blood centers, but also any entity that engages in the manufacturing of blood products, including establishments that test blood donations and those whose products are used in the blood-manufacturing process. These counts are at the establishment level (not unique organizations). In Figure 2.2, we present total counts of unique blood establishments by health care market (defined in Chapter Three).

Next, we describe the main stakeholders in the U.S. blood system:

Donors: Typically unpaid, donors are screened and then donate either whole blood or specific blood components (through apheresis). As noted earlier, we focus on volunteer donors (for whole blood) instead of paid plasma donors. Plasma collection is different in several ways that make its cost of production significantly lower: Plasma can be frozen and thus stored or transported for longer periods of time, more safely, and less expensively; and donors can donate plasma more frequently (twice a week

Figure 2.1
Number of Blood Establishments Registered with FDA, by Facility Type and Geographic Region

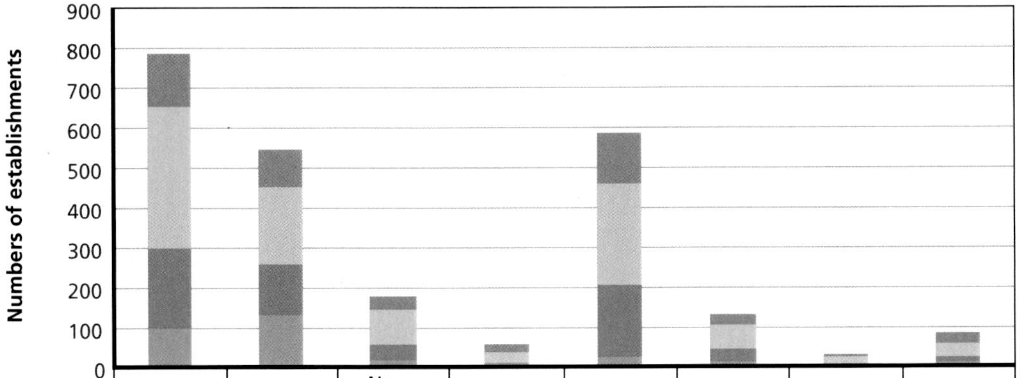

	Collection	Hospital blood banks	Non-hospital blood banks	Ware-house	Processing	Distribu-tion	Testing	Other
West	132	88	37	17	125	27	6	26
South	356	200	86	28	253	60	17	33
Midwest	198	121	40	1	182	32	3	15
Northeast	100	134	18	12	24	12	2	12

SOURCE: Form 2830 data provided by the FDA, 2016. See Chapter Three for a description of these data.
RAND RR1575-2.1

versus once every eight weeks) and can donate significantly more per donation.[1] However, plasma donation takes longer (two hours versus ten minutes for a whole blood draw).

Blood centers: Blood collection centers are typically nonprofit organizations committed to collecting and supplying blood in their communities. Following industry practice, we use the term *blood center* to refer to corporate entities even when the entity has multiple physical collection, processing, distribution, and research locations. The largest single blood center—the American Red Cross (ARC)—operates many collection locations. Other independent blood centers belong to consortia, such as America's Blood Centers (ABC). Blood centers sometimes provide other services—for example, blood-related research, organ donor matching, blood testing, and information technology (IT) services—and could fit into other categories listed in this section. While increasingly rare, some hospitals internally run their own blood centers.

Suppliers and other blood establishments: Blood centers rely on goods and services from a range of suppliers, including consumables like bags used in blood collection, blood testing and typing, inventory and tracking systems, and logistics.

---

[1]   Slonim, Wang, and Garbarino, 2014.

Figure 2.2
Number of Unique Blood Establishments Registered with FDA, per Hospital Referral Region

- ■ (8,33]
- ■ (4,8]
- ▨ (2,4]
- ▢ (1,2]
- ▢ (0,1]

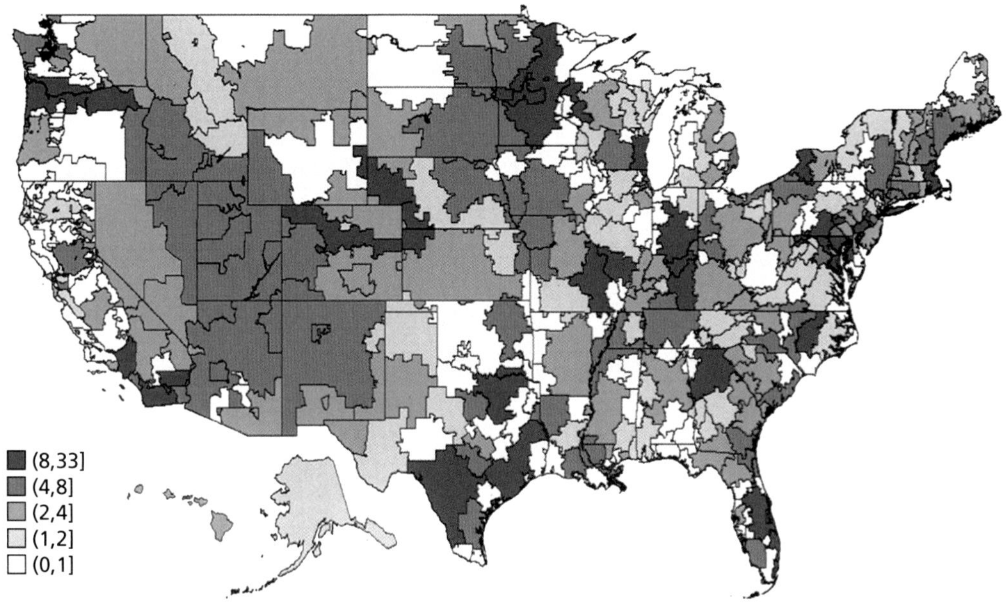

SOURCE: RAND analysis of FDA Form 2830 data by hospital referral region (HRR). See Chapter Three for more details.

RAND RR1575-2.2

Hospitals: Hospitals and health systems deliver the bulk of health care services requiring blood, including surgery, trauma care, treatments for some cancers, organ transplantation procedures, obstetrical bleeding, and numerous acute and chronic anemic conditions, including blood disorders. Hospitals in the United States are increasingly integrating with other hospitals and broader health care systems. Although increasingly rare, some hospitals also run their own blood collection facilities that fill a portion of their facilities' blood needs. Most hospitals acquire blood entirely from external sources. Hospital transfusion services, typically called "blood banks," acquire, store, compatibility match, and distribute blood components for patient use.

Clinicians: Clinicians—including practitioners specializing in transfusion medicine, oncology, surgery, and a range of other areas—and their clinical support staff, decide whether and how to use blood, provide a range of other health care services (some of which are reliant on blood), transfuse blood, and monitor patients.

Payers: Payers, including large public payers, such as Medicare and state Medicaid programs and private insurers, compensate hospitals for the care that they deliver to patients. They rarely—if ever—pay blood centers directly. For inpatient care (e.g., hospital stays), most payers use a bundled payment approach in which hospitals receive the same amount per stay regardless of whether or how blood is used.

FDA: FDA is responsible for regulating biological and related products, including blood and blood components. FDA's regulatory oversight is aimed at ensuring the safety, potency, and purity of blood and blood components by promulgating regulations and guidance for the collection, testing, processing, storage, and transport of blood and blood components. FDA may seek external expert scientific advice relevant to regulation through the Blood Products Advisory Committee.

Centers for Disease Control and Prevention (CDC): CDC contributes blood-related research, surveillance, and prevention activities related to blood-borne pathogens. CDC also contributes to and hosts the United States' only nationwide hemovigilance (HV) reporting system, which endeavors to track transfusion-related adverse events.

National Institutes of Health (NIH): NIH, including the National Heart, Lung, and Blood Institute (NHLBI), funds intramural and extramural research conducted at blood centers, universities, and other organizations. For example, in 2012, NHLBI grants related to blood research totaled more than $400 million. NIH's support of clinical research influences blood usage, such as establishing target hematocrit levels or researching substitutes for blood products.[2]

Office of the Assistant Secretary for Preparedness and Response (ASPR) and Biomedical Advanced Research and Development Authority (BARDA): HHS ASPR, in addition to broad responsibilities related to preparedness, coordinates BARDA, which makes investments into translational and clinical research for a range of biodefense and other technologies, including blood technologies.

U.S. Department of Defense (DoD): DoD has a separate blood collection system for the military health care system, military personnel, and their beneficiaries, which is partially integrated with the broader U.S. blood system. Collectively, the ASBP operates more than 20 blood centers and 61 transfusion services entities.[3] The ASBP collects blood from service members, beneficiaries, and civilians,[4] but it is limited to collecting blood on military and federal installations.[5] However, civilian agencies can collect blood on military installations through written agreement.[6] DoD also funds a significant volume of blood-related research in the fields of trauma care, blood-product innovation, and pathogen reduction technology (PRT).

The U.S. Department of Veterans Affairs (VA): VA and the Veterans Health Administration's (VHA's) blood establishment network sometimes use blood provided

---

[2]   NHLBI, "NHLBI Blood Diseases and Resources Program: Obligations by Funding Mechanism, Fiscal Year 2012," 2012.

[3]   ASBP, *ASBP Educational Campaign Fact Sheet*, Falls Church, Va., 2015b.

[4]   ASBP, home page, 2015f.

[5]   DoD, *Department of Defense Instruction 6480.04: Armed Services Blood Program Operational Procedures*, Washington, D.C., 2013.

[6]   ASBP, 2015f.

Figure 2.3
Overview of Blood Collection and Utilization in the United States

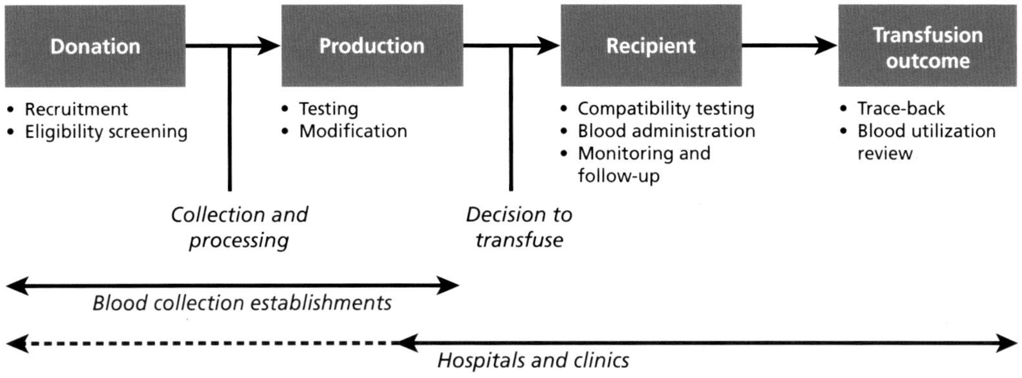

SOURCE: Adapted from AABB (formerly known as the American Association of Blood Banks).
RAND RR1575-2.3

by the ASBP. VA and VHA operated at least 15 hospital blood banks and 60 hospital transfusion centers throughout the United States in 2015,[7] and, according to one VA official, they currently operate 134 hospital blood banks/transfusion services and no donor centers.

Vein-to-Vein Process

The following sections describe how the stakeholders just defined interact and key processes, as outlined in Figure 2.3, at four stages: donation, production, recipient, and transfusion outcome.

Donation

Blood donation can be for anonymous use by others (allogeneic), for one's own use in which a patient's own blood is processed and retransfused (autologous), or for a family or friend's use, typically in anticipation of an upcoming procedure (directed). Donors can provide blood both without compensation (volunteer) and with compensation (especially for plasma), as defined by FDA regulations.[8]

In the United States, blood is collected from donors by a wide range of blood establishments, all of which must be registered and licensed by FDA. Blood establish-

---

[7]   FDA, "Blood Establishment Registration Database," updated as of January 8, 2016a.

[8]   World Health Organization (WHO), *Global Database on Blood Safety: Summary Report 2011*, Geneva, Switzerland: World Health Organization, 2011b; U.S. National Library of Medicine, "Blood Donation Before Surgery," 2015; Bruce Newman, "Blood Donor Suitability and Allogeneic Whole Blood Donation," *Transfusion Medicine Reviews,* Vol. 15, No. 3, 2001, pp. 234–244; ABC, "Types of Blood Donations," undated-b; ARC, home page, undated-a.

ments engaging in interstate distribution are required to obtain additional licensing. As of 2016 (see Figure 2.1), there were nearly 786 registered blood establishments that collect blood (plus an additional 725 hospital and nonhospital blood banks), with blood centers collecting 93 percent of allogeneic whole blood and hospital blood banks collecting about 7 percent of allogeneic whole blood.[9] Blood for autologous and directed use comprised about 1 percent of all blood units collected in 2011.[10]

Recruitment and Screening

All people who donate blood for human use in the United States must be screened per FDA regulations and must meet certain eligibility requirements, which can depend on the type and intended use of the blood product.[11] In addition, certain organizations or establishments can implement additional standards or guidelines that are specific to populations, programs, type of blood product, and use.

Donors who do not meet minimum requirements, as ascertained from an FDA-accepted Donor History Questionnaire or similar standardized screening material developed by AABB[12] or the Plasma Protein Therapeutics Association,[13] will be deferred or not allowed to donate blood for a period of time. The period of time for which the donor is deferred varies based on the predicted risk to the donor, the recipient, or both.

Collection

The main blood components include red blood cells (RBCs), platelets, granulocytes, and plasma, all of which are prepared and manufactured using either whole blood donations or apheresis.[14] Whole blood donations are used most commonly for RBC and plasma products and require subsequent processing steps to separate RBCs from white cells, plasma, and platelets.[15] Apheresis, the use of a medical apparatus to collect only a specific blood component from a donor, is used to produce 75 percent of platelet

---

[9]   Authors' analysis of FDA data (see Chapter Three).

[10]   Chung et al., 2016.

[11]   FDA, Food and Drugs, Code of Federal Regulations, Title 21, Part 640.3, Suitability of Donor, 1999.

[12]   FDA, "Changes to an Approved Application: Biological Products: Human Blood and Blood Components Intended for Transfusion or for Further Manufacture: Guidance for Industry," Center for Biologics Evaluation and Research, December 2014b; FDA, "Recommendations for Assessment of Blood Donor Suitability, Donor Deferral and Blood Product Management in Response to Ebola Virus: Draft Guidance for Industry," Center for Biologics Evaluation and Research, December 2015b.

[13]   Plasma Protein Therapeutics Association, home page, undated; FDA, "Implementation of Acceptable Full-Length and Abbreviated Donor History Questionnaires and Accompanying Materials for Use in Screening Donors of Source Plasma: Guidance for Industry," July 2016b.

[14]   Mark Fung, Brenda Grossman, Christopher Hillyer, and Connie Westhoff, *AABB Technical Manual*, 18th ed., 2014.

[15]   ARC, "Types of Donations," undated-b.

products in the United States.[16] During a platelet donation, an apheresis machine collects platelets while returning RBCs and most plasma to the donor.[17] Donor burden (donation time and other requirements), as well as collection costs, can be higher with apheresis. The plasma collection system for manufacturing of derivatives is mostly separate from the whole blood collection system.

Production
Processing
Like drugs regulated by FDA, blood and components are collected and processed under current Good Manufacturing Practices (GMP). Post-collection processing mostly involves separating whole blood collections into individual blood components (RBCs, plasma, cryoprecipitate, platelets) within eight hours of donation. With apheresis, component separation happens during collection because apheresis removes individual blood components.

RBCs and platelets derived from whole blood are generally filtered for leukocyte removal, to mitigate the buildup of cytokines and other inflammatory molecules that can lead to adverse reactions and to prevent transmission of some cell-associated viruses, such as cytomegalovirus. In 2013, 72 percent of all whole blood and RBC units were leuko-reduced in the United States.[18] Plasma is what remains after platelets, white blood cells, and RBCs have been removed.

Other procedures that can occur at the processing stage include freezing blood and blood components and irradiation.[19] The processing of blood also includes packaging it into a variety of bag configurations and sizes to accommodate various patient needs, including small aliquots for pediatric use. Finally, processing blood and blood components involves ensuring the proper disposal of the medical waste generated during processing. In addition, expired blood and components are labeled, tracked, and often used for research.[20]

Testing
There are two main types of tests necessary before blood components are suitable for human use: testing for infectious diseases and testing to match the blood type of the donor to the recipient (blood-typing, antibodies, and more).

---

[16] ARC, undated-b.

[17] ARC, undated-b.

[18] Chung et al., 2016.

[19] Cost of Blood Consensus Conference, "The Cost of Blood: Multidisciplinary Consensus Conference for a Standard Methodology," *Transfusion Medicine Reviews*, Vol. 19, No. 1, January 2005, pp. 66–78; American Association for Clinical Chemistry, "Transfusion Medicine," December 3, 2015.

[20] Cost of Blood Consensus Conference, 2015.

FDA requires "one or more such tests as necessary to reduce adequately and appropriately the risk of transmission of communicable disease."[21] Current FDA regulations require all blood donations to be tested for specific infectious agents, including syphilis, human immunodeficiency virus (HIV) type 1 and type 2, hepatitis B virus (HBV), hepatitis C virus (HCV), and human T-cell lymphotropic virus type I and type II. A final rule issued in May 2015 (effective May 2016) requires donor eligibility screening for risks of variant Creutzfeld-Jakob disease and malaria and tests for additional pathogens, including West Nile virus and the agent of Chagas disease. Many centers already test for these agents. Guidelines have also been developed to recommend testing for certain agents as they arise as potential threats to the blood supply, including dengue, babesia, and bacterial contamination. In February 2016, FDA also approved a Zika virus screening test for investigational use, and some labs began testing all blood for Zika at that time.[22] Testing of donated blood is now largely conducted at centralized laboratories that can capitalize on high-throughput automation and minimize human error.[23]

Modification

Screening and testing alone cannot exclude all potential human pathogens. Therefore, PRTs involving physical, chemical, or photochemical approaches unselectively inactivate infectious agents in the blood. PRTs can also preclude the need for some testing. However, any strategy that involves additives or physical manipulation of blood must balance the benefits of pathogen reduction (PR) against the loss or damage to the cells and plasma proteins, potential toxicity to the recipient, financial cost, potential contamination of the environment, and risk to the personnel involved in the process. Currently, there is one FDA-approved PRT for platelets, and there are two FDA-approved PRTs for plasma.

Logistics and Inventory Management

Beyond testing and processing, blood ready for transfusion has to be transported, stored, and inventoried prior to use. FDA also regulates blood storage requirements to ensure safety throughout its life cycle (see the appendix for more details).

---

[21] FDA, 2015a.

[22] *Newsweek* magazine (see Jessica Firger, "FDA Approves First Zika Diagnostic Test for Commercial Use," *Newsweek*, February 26, 2016) and a supplier interview mentioned that labs began testing all of their blood for Zika in February 2016.

[23] J. F. Quaranta, F. Berthier, R. Courbil, F. Courtois, F. Chenais, C. Waller, M. F. Leconte des Floris, G. Andreu, O. Fontaine, C. Le Niger, M. Puntous, A. Mercadier, L. Nguyen, E. Pelissier, G. Gondrexon, and P. Staccini., "Qui sont les receveurs de produits sanguins labiles (PSL)? Une étude nationale multicentrique—un jour donné. Établissement de transfusion sanguine (ETS)—établissements de santé (ES) [Who are the recipients of labile blood products? A Multicenter Nationwide Study—A 'Donation Day.' Blood Banks, Health Facilities], *Transfusion Clinique et Biologique: Journal de la Societe Francaise de Transfusion Sanguine*, Vol. 16. No. 1, pp. 21–29.

Blood would need to be discarded prior to transfusion because of the following factors: (1) expiration (units exceeding their licensed shelf life, which varies by blood component), (2) lack of temperature control (units moved out of refrigeration exceeding a defined period of time cannot be returned to main stock, (3) refrigerator failure (e.g., due to power outage, equipment malfunction), and (4) other miscellaneous problems (e.g., dropping a unit of blood, damaging its packaging).[24] According to the National Blood Collection and Utilization Survey (NBCUS), the blood components outdated by blood centers and hospitals were 306,000 units in 2013 (95 percent confidence interval 269,000 to 343,000), which represented approximately 2.3 percent of all collected units.[25] The 2013 NBCUS does not separately report units wasted for other reasons. However, the 2011 survey reported 233,330 wasted units, which represented 0.8 percent of all collected units (this rate likely varies by blood type, although separate statistics by type are not collected in NBCUS).[26] Given its shorter shelf life of five to seven days, wastage of platelets is generally higher than wastage of other blood components.[27]

Recipient

Hospital Administration and Processes

Hospitals and blood centers face significant challenges in blood inventory management. They must balance the need to carry sufficient stock to fulfill both anticipated and unanticipated demands for blood and minimize waste at the same time. Poor inventory management practices are costly for centers and hospitals, as well as the larger health system.[28] Within hospitals, blood demand tends to be forecasted based on historical patterns of use.[29] To facilitate inventory management, hospitals rely on a variety of tools, including staff expertise, internal inventory management software, external inventory management that blood centers provide, or all three.

---

[24] S. H. Stanger, N. Yates, R. Wilding, and S. Cotton, "Blood Inventory Management: Hospital Best Practice," *Transfusion Medicine Reviews*, Vol. 26, No. 2, April 2012, pp. 153–163.

[25] Chung et al., 2016.

[26] HHS, *The 2011 National Blood Collection and Utilization Survey Report*, Washington, D.C.: U.S. Department of Health and Human Services, 2011b.

[27] HHS, 2011b.

[28] Stanger et al., 2012.

[29] Lorna M. Williamson and Dana V. Devine, "Challenges in the Management of the Blood Supply," *Lancet*, Vol. 381, No. 9880, May 25, 2013, pp. 1866–1875.

Use of Blood by U.S. Hospitals

According to the 2011 NBCUS, the total number of all blood components transfused in 2011 was 20,933,000, a decrease of 11.6 percent from 2008.[30] The vast majority of transfusions occur in hospitals. Transfusions occur in more than 10 percent of all hospitalizations that include a procedure,[31] and 5 percent to 8 percent of all hospital discharges are associated with a blood transfusion.[32] While the vast majority of blood components are transfused in acute care hospitals, other settings for transfusions include physician offices, dialysis centers, home health agencies, and skilled nursing facilities (SNFs).[33] In this report, we focus exclusively on the use of blood by hospitals because they are the chief setting for transfusions.

Within the hospital, the services that use the greatest quantities of RBCs include general medicine (31 percent), surgery (20 percent), and hematology and oncology (15 percent). In contrast, the services with the greatest use of platelet products are hematology and oncology (34 percent), surgery (18 percent), general medicine (17 percent), and intensive care units (ICUs) (12 percent). [34]

Transfusion Outcome

Adverse Events and Complications of Transfusions

The justification for hospital patient blood management programs to minimize the medically unnecessary use of blood, as well as the general approach by hospitals and clinicians to avoid using blood components where possible, is that transfusions are not without risk to patients. In fact, blood transfusions have been described as "unsafe" and "inherently dangerous" in U.S. Blood Shield laws.[35] The probability of an adverse reaction, although small, should be factored into any decision to order a transfusion. In addition, frequent transfusions might also be linked to poorer outcomes, including increased patient mortality, a higher incidence of nosocomial infections and multior-

---

[30] HHS, 2011b.

[31] L. T. Goodnough, "Blood Management: Transfusion Medicine Comes of Age," *Lancet*, Vol. 381, No. 9880, May 25, 2013, pp. 1791–1792.

[32] L. T. Goodnough, J. H. Levy, and M. F. Murphy, "Concepts of Blood Transfusion in Adults," *Lancet*, Vol. 381, No. 9880, May 25, 2013, pp. 1845–1854; J. Macpherson, C. B. Mahoney, L. Katz, J. Haarmann, and C. Bianco, "Contribution of Blood to Hospital Revenue in the United States," *Transfusion*, Vol. 47, No. 2, Supplement, August 2007, pp. 114S–116S, discussion pp. 117S–119S.

[33] C. Goodman, S. Chan, P. Collins, R. Haught, and Y. J. Chen, "Ensuring Blood Safety and Availability in the U.S.: Technological Advances, Costs, and Challenges to Payment—Final Report," *Transfusion*, Vol. 43, No. 8, Supplement, August 2003, pp. 3s–46s.

[34] HHS, 2011b.

[35] Goodnough, 2013.

gan failure, and increased length of hospital and ICU stays.[36] Identifying these links empirically is difficult because sicker individuals tend to be more likely to receive transfusions, receive more units of blood in a transfusion, and stay longer in hospitals.

According to NBCUS, 50,570 adverse reactions were reported to hospital transfusion services in 2011, which is likely an underestimate of all transfusion-related adverse reactions.[37] Out of these, approximately 21,000 were severe. According to these data, the adverse reaction rate (adverse reactions and total components transfused) has remained fairly constant over time: In 2011, it was 0.24 percent, a negligible decrease from 0.25 percent in 2008 and 0.26 percent in 2006.[38] The most common adverse reactions in transfusions in 2011 in the United States were fever (43 percent), allergic reactions (28 percent), and delayed serologic transfusion reactions (5 percent).

Payment for Blood, Transfusion Services, and Other Health Care Services Involving Blood

While blood centers are paid by hospitals that purchase blood, health insurers reimburse hospitals and other entities that perform transfusions. Approximately 92 percent to 95 percent of blood is transfused in the inpatient setting.[39] Medicare is the dominant payer for inpatient hospital services, and 46 percent of patients who receive blood-intensive procedures, such as transplants, are Medicare beneficiaries.[40]

Medicare and most private payers reimburse for hospital-inpatient care under the diagnosis-related groups (DRGs) prospective payment system. DRGs are assigned based on a patient's primary and secondary diagnoses and the procedures performed during the inpatient stay. Hospitals receive a fixed, prospectively determined payment for each DRG, regardless of actual services rendered. As such, costs associated with blood and blood components are rolled into some DRGs, and reimbursement stays the same regardless of which (and how many) blood components are transfused into a particular patient or which or how many transfusion-related services are delivered.[41]

Payment for blood and transfusions in the outpatient setting is somewhat different. CMS now reimburses hospitals under the hospital Outpatient Prospective Payment System (OPPS) with different prospectively determined payment rates for individual ambulatory payment classification (APC) categories. In this system, cases are assigned to APC groups based on Current Procedural Terminology (CPT) diagnosis

---

[36] Aryeh Shander, Axel Hofmann, Hans Gombotz, Oliver M. Theusinger, and Donat R. Spahn, "Estimating the Cost of Blood: Past, Present, and Future Directions," *Best Practice and Research Clinical Anaesthesiology*, Vol. 21, No. 2, June 2007, pp. 271–289.

[37] Chung et al., 2016.

[38] HHS, 2011b.

[39] Goodman et al., 2003.

[40] Goodman et al., 2003.

[41] AABB, *AABB Billing Guide for Transfusion and Cellular Therapy Services*, Bethesda, Md., October 2007.

codes and Healthcare Common Procedure Coding System (HCPCS) procedure codes. Transfused blood and blood products are uniquely reimbursed separately under their own APCs. In contrast with what happens in inpatient DRGs, transfused blood and blood products in outpatient settings are not rolled into the APC payment associated with the procedures provided.[42]

Surveillance and Public Health

In addition to the system for collecting, processing, and dispensing blood, there is a public health apparatus that (1) monitors the outcomes of these activities and uses the information to improve patient safety and (2) has responsibility for ensuring the availability of blood in the event of a public health crisis.

Biovigilance and Surveillance

HHS's Advisory Committee on Blood and Tissue Safety and Availability has defined *biovigilance* as a "comprehensive and integrated national patient safety program to collect, analyze and report on the outcomes of collection and transfusion or transplantation of blood components and derivatives, cells, tissues, and organs," and it has recommended biovigilance as a systemwide effort to improve patient safety. Biovigilance specific to transfusion-related adverse events is referred to as HV. Although national HV systems are well established in most developed countries, AABB's U.S. Biovigilance Network and CDC only recently began to establish a nationwide, centralized repository of HV data: the HV Module of the National Healthcare Safety Network (NHSN).[43] This HV Module is a surveillance system designed to monitor patients' and health care workers' safety. Some hospitals use this tool to monitor adverse events associated with blood transfusions at the local and national levels, but the United States has no central organization tasked with monitoring or analyzing these data.[44] Participation in this program is voluntary and passive—only some hospitals participate, and the system depends on staff to take the initiative to report adverse transfusion-related events.[45]

AABB's Donor Hemovigilance Analysis and Reporting Tool is used to track and reduce the occurrence of adverse events associated with blood donation.[46] The program relies on hospital and blood center reporting, which is analyzed to generate facility-specific reports and benchmarks and can then be aggregated to identify trends. Par-

---

[42]   AABB, 2007.

[43]   CDC, NHSN, "Blood Safety Surveillance," last updated September 2016.

[44]   HHS, *Biovigilance in the United States: Efforts to Bridge a Critical Gap in Patient Safety and Donor Health*, Washington, D.C.: HHS, 2009.

[45]   CDC, NHSN, "Frequently Asked Questions About Hemovigilance Module," last updated February 2016.

[46]   AABB, "Donor Hemovigilance," undated-b.

ticipation in the program requires an annual fee, adoption of standard definitions for donor reaction, and reporting of adverse events.

Despite these systems, there are concerns regarding several gaps in HV, including a fragmented system of adverse event reporting with underreporting and concerns about accuracy. U.S. HV also lacks national surveillance of donors' serious adverse events other than reporting of fatalities to FDA. However, a national program to track donor infectious disease test data from more than 50 percent of collections was established recently.[47] FDA intends to finalize a regulation that will mandate reporting of serious adverse reactions to blood donation and blood transfusion.[48]

Preparedness and Response

Emerging infectious agents and natural disasters are examples of public health risks, as well as potential disruptions to the supply and demand for blood. Thus, regular systemwide monitoring of the supply and demand of blood is imperative to ensure the safety and availability of blood. There is no single, national U.S. system, but rather there are various entities and systems in place to manage such risks and monitor the supply and demand of blood from different angles:

- OASH at HHS is the safety officer, as authorized by the National Response Framework for Emergency Support Function.[49] OASH works with other agencies, including the Health Resources and Services Administration (HRSA), CDC, NIH, FDA, CMS, and the Agency for Healthcare Research and Quality to coordinate all public health issues concerning blood.
- AABB's Interorganizational Task Force on Domestic Disasters and Acts of Terrorism (hereafter referred to as the Task Force),[50] established in January 2002, coordinates response efforts (e.g., collection, transportation, communication to the public) for domestic disasters or acts of terrorism. The Task Force includes AABB members and liaisons from HHS, CDC, FDA, and ASBP.
- There are additional tools for local blood centers and hospitals to monitor the supply and demand of blood, including tracking by ABC and the Blood Availability and Safety Information System (BASIS),[51] which allows users to gather and analyze blood collection and usage information from hospitals and blood centers across the United States.

---

[47] FDA, " Blood Products Advisory Committee Meeting Issue Summary," 111th Meeting, December 2, 2014c.

[48] FDA, 2015a.

[49] Federal Emergency Management Agency, "Emergency Support Function No. 8—Public Health and Medical Services Annex," January 2008.

[50] AABB, "Disaster Response," undated-a.

[51] Knowledge Based Systems, Inc., "Blood Availability & Safety Information System (BASIS)," undated.

- The National Blood Exchange (NBE) is an AABB program established for blood sharing. The NBE system provides blood centers a mechanism through which surplus blood may be moved to areas in need and provides hospitals with additional blood if their current supply cannot meet anticipated needs.
- FDA (effective September 8, 2015)[52] requires licensed applicants of blood and blood components for transfusion that manufacture at least 10 percent or more of the U.S. blood supply,[53] among others, to notify FDA about certain discontinuances or disruptions to the supply for blood and blood components. This rule is intended to inform FDA of potential shortages that could help FDA predict and manage or mitigate large-scale or nationwide disruptions in the U.S. blood supply.
- Internationally, WHO maintains the Global Database on Blood Safety,[54] which provides information on global blood collection, donation, infrastructure, blood screening, blood processing, and use of blood collected from questionnaires sent to national health authorities.

---

[52] HHS, "Permanent Discontinuance or Interruption in Manufacturing of Certain Drug or Biological Products," *Federal Register*, Vol. 80, No. 130, July 8, 2015.

[53] Based on the 2011 NBCUS data, 10 percent or more of the U.S. blood supply would mean more than 1.5 million units of whole blood annually or approximately 125,000 units per month. At the time the rule was passed, FDA estimated that the rule affected 411 different establishments under four separate licenses.

[54] WHO, "Global Database on Blood Safety," undated.

CHAPTER THREE

Methods

In this chapter, we outline the overall analytic approach for this study, with a focus on describing qualitative and quantitative data and methods used across several chapters. Chapters Four through Nine contain additional notes on these methods where appropriate. Broadly, we employ a mixed-methods approach in which we blend qualitative analysis with available quantitative evidence and empirics.

Qualitative Approach

Our primary qualitative data sources were semi-structured telephone interviews and focus groups with key blood system stakeholders. We interviewed representatives from ten blood centers, eight hospitals, and 11 corporations that supply equipment and services to blood centers and hospitals (hereafter referred to as "suppliers") from February to June 2016. We had separate conversations with CDC, CMS, FDA, HHS, NIH, and OASH blood experts over the same time period.

Our reliance on interviews with organizations that together currently comprise the U.S. blood system could cause us to emphasize the benefits of maintaining the status quo. We have attempted to compensate for this inherent bias by balancing industry perspectives with outsider perspectives, including our own.

Blood Centers
We selected the blood centers from a list of possible candidates provided by HHS and ABC. We asked ABC to provide a list of candidates that represented the full diversity of the industry, and we selected centers from this list to ensure diversity in terms of geographic location and size (as measured by annual units of blood collected).

We invited ten blood centers to participate using maximum variation sampling, and nine accepted and participated in a telephone interview for a response rate of 90 percent (see Table 3.1). For one of these nine blood centers, we interviewed two leaders. Six of these blood center leaders were chief executive officers, one was a director of sales, one was a chief operating officer, one was a senior adviser, and one was an

Table 3.1
Participating Blood Centers

Blood Center	Census Region	Relative Blood Center Size
1	South	Small
2	West	Small
3	South	Small
4	South	Medium
5	West, Northeast	Medium
6	Midwest	Medium
7	Midwest	Large
8	National	Large
9	National	Large

NOTE: Small blood centers collect 75,000 or fewer units per year; medium-sized centers collect 75,001 to 200,000 units per year; and large blood centers collect 200,001 or more units per year.

executive vice president. We also interviewed one medical doctor running a hospital-based center (not reflected in the earlier tallies or in Table 3.1).

We conducted one-hour, semi-structured interviews with each of the 11 leaders. Interviews followed a detailed protocol, including questions on health care system trends affecting the industry and the likely effects of those trends on blood center operations. At least one RAND researcher and a research assistant who took notes were present at each interview.

We also conducted two in-person focus groups on March 12, 2016, at the ABC annual meeting. Each focus group lasted 60 minutes and included four blood center leaders and two RAND facilitators. Focus groups consisted of the same blood center leaders who participated in telephone interviews. The focus groups allowed blood center leaders to elaborate on their previous observations and publicly compare and contrast their perspectives with others in their industry. The focus groups also provided the study team with an opportunity to ask follow-up questions and clarify some of the answers given during the earlier telephone interviews.

Hospitals

As with blood centers, we interviewed a diverse group of hospital representatives. We assembled a convenience sample through snowball sampling and organizational connections. We asked the blood centers that participated in interviews to provide the contact information of two or more hospitals that they supply, and we selected several hospitals from these referrals. We also independently reached out to several hospitals within our research networks to obtain maximum variation on hospital size and geography.

Of the 39 hospital transfusion experts referred to us by HHS, blood centers, hospitals, and other RAND contacts, we invited ten hospitals with at least some regular level of blood transfusion activity to participate in interviews. Eight of these ten hospital representatives completed phone interviews for a response rate of 80 percent (see Table 3.2). Participating hospital representatives included directors of transfusions and directors of laboratory services and operations. One of the participating hospital representatives was a manager of a hospital-owned blood bank. Five of the hospitals we interviewed were part of a large academic medical center or system.

As with blood centers, we conducted one-hour, semi-structured interviews with each of the hospital representatives, following a detailed protocol with questions on the relationships between blood centers and hospitals, health care trends, and other topics (see the appendix for the interview protocol).

Suppliers

We interviewed organizations that supply hospitals and blood centers with various goods and services. These suppliers sell medical devices, including blood-manufacturing equipment, transportation services, blood testing services and equipment, consulting services, and blood sales platforms.

Some of the companies that manufacture and sell products, devices, and equipment to collect, process, and test blood are represented by the AdvaMed trade association, which helped facilitate and anonymize some written interview responses. By networking with representatives of AdvaMed and other suppliers who volunteered to talk with us on the sidelines of the ABC 2016 annual meeting, by cold-calling one group

Table 3.2
Participating Hospitals

U.S. Census Region	Number of Beds	Number of Hospitals Within Network or System
Midwest	<500	1
South	<500	2–5
Northeast	<500	1
Northeast	>500	>5
Northeast	>1,000	>5
Midwest	<500	2–5
Midwest	>500	1
West	<500	1

purchasing organization (GPO), and by asking our blood center and GPO contacts for introductions to blood exchanges, we were able to identify and interview seven equipment manufacturers, one blood testing service, one GPO, and two blood exchanges.

As with hospitals and blood centers, we conducted one-hour, semi-structured interviews with four of the aforementioned equipment manufacturing leaders. Interviews followed a detailed protocol that included questions on trends affecting the industry and the likely effects of those trends on manufacturer sales, prices, and investments in R&D (see the appendix for the interview protocol). At least one RAND researcher and a research assistant who took notes were present at each interview. Three additional managers of blood-related equipment manufacturers answered similar written questions that AdvaMed forwarded to them. AdvaMed informed us that at least three of their members contributed anonymously to our email interview, and it was not clear how many declined. All of these suppliers also answered follow-up questions via email to clarify or expand on their interview responses, and one of them also spoke with us via a one-hour telephone interview.

In addition to telephone and email interviews with device and equipment suppliers, we also conducted one-hour telephone interviews with managers of organizations that supply blood testing services, consulting, and market exchange services.

Government Regulators and Other Stakeholders

We interviewed U.S. government agencies and departments that support or regulate the U.S. blood system. This included one-hour telephone interviews with officials from the FDA Center for Biologics Evaluation and Research (CBER), HHS's ASPR, BARDA, and NIH. We also discussed FDA data and the NBCUS with individuals at FDA and CDC, respectively (see details on these data sources in the next section).

Quantitative Analyses

We relied primarily on previous empirical studies. However, in the following sections, we briefly highlight three key data sources used to inform multiple chapters in this report. In cases where we used unique data for only one chapter, we include these details in the corresponding chapter. We explored analyzing 990 tax data to examine costs in the blood supply chain more carefully but found that granular cost reporting was inconsistent and measured at differing organizational levels (e.g., ARC) making it difficult to analyze costs specific to blood collection consistently across organizations.

National Blood Collection and Utilization Survey

The NBCUS has been fielded approximately biennially since 2004, and it is sponsored by several divisions within HHS—CDC, CMS, FDA, HRSA, and NIH. In previous years, the survey was fielded by AABB. However, in 2013, CDC collected the data.

The sampling frame for the NBCUS has been derived from FDA Form 2830, which all regulated blood establishments are required to submit annually to FDA. The NBCUS was sent to blood centers, hospitals, cord blood banks, and other blood establishment entities, but these organizations might not be representative of all types of establishments. The NBCUS survey instrument contains rich data related to blood transfusions, processes, and practices.

We were unable to obtain the underlying microdata for this report, but we drew on aggregated statistics presented in the 2005, 2007, 2009, 2011, and 2013 reports.[1] We used these data to describe trends in the cost of blood, but we note that the data are dated.

CMS Data

We analyzed CMS's After Outliers Removed (AOR)/Before Outliers Removed (BOR) File from the 2016 Inpatient Prospective Payment System Final Rule, as described in Chapter Five.

FDA Form 2830 Data Linked to Dartmouth Atlas Market Level Data

To describe the distribution of the different types of establishments across the United States, we used FDA Form 2830, which all regulated blood establishments are required to provide annually to the FDA.[2] We also merged these data with hospital- and market-level data from the Dartmouth Atlas, which is derived from fee-for-service Medicare claims data, census (population) data, and the data from the Area Health Resource File.[3] We defined the health care market by HRR.[4] We used Dartmouth Atlas data from 2012 (the most recent year consistently available). Next, we describe the measures used and calculated from each data set.

---

[1]   HHS, *The 2005 National Blood Collection and Utilization Survey Report*, Washington, D.C.: HHS, OASH, 2005; HHS, *The 2007 National Blood Collection and Utilization Survey Report*, Washington, D.C.: HHS, OASH, 2007; HHS, *The 2009 National Blood Collection and Utilization Survey Report*, Washington, D.C.: HHS, OASH, 2011a; Chung et al., 2011; and HHS, *The 2013 National Blood Collection and Utilization Survey Report*, Washington, D.C.: HHS, OASH, 2013.

[2]   FDA, Establishment Registration and Product Listing for Manufactures of Human Blood and Blood Products, Title 21, Code of Federal Regulations, Part 607, undated.

[3]   D. C. Goodman, A. Esty, E. S. Fisher, and C. H. Chang, "A Report of the Dartmouth Atlas Project," Hanover, N.H.: The Dartmouth Institute for Health Policy and Clinical Practice, 2010, p. 37; D. C. Goodman, E. S. Fisher, C. H. Chang, S. R. Raymond, and K. K. Bronner, "After Hospitalization: A Dartmouth Atlas Report on Post-Acute Care for Medicare Beneficiaries," Hanover, N.H.: The Dartmouth Institute for Health Policy and Clinical Practice, Vol. 28, 2011.

[4]   J. E. Wennberg, "Appendix on the Geography of Health Care in the United States," *The Dartmouth Atlas of Health Care in the United States*, 1990, pp. 289–296.

- **FDA Form 2830 Data**
  - Counts of all blood establishments and by facility type—collection, nonhospital or community blood bank, hospital blood bank, hospital transfusion service, broker or warehouse, processing (includes plasmapheresis and component preparation), distribution, testing, and others
- **Dartmouth Atlas**
  - Hospital Level
    ◦ Counts of hospitals in each HRR
    ◦ Number of inpatient discharges annually in each HRR
    ◦ Hospital Herfindahl-Hirschman Index (HHI)—calculated as the sum of the market shares squared for each hospital in the HRR and ranges from 0 to 1, where a larger value represents a more highly concentrated market. For example, an HRR with ten hospitals with equal shares of the market ($HHI = 10 \times 0.1^2 = 0.1$) is less concentrated (more competitive) than a market with two hospitals with equal shares of the market ($HHI = 0.5^2 + 0.5^2 = 0.5$). We defined share of the market as equal to the number of Medicare inpatient discharges at each hospital divided by the total number of Medicare inpatient discharges in the HRR.
  - Market Level
    ◦ Population (2010 data)
    ◦ Acute care hospital beds per 1,000 residents
    ◦ Hospital-based registered nurses per 1,000 residents
    ◦ Full-time equivalent (FTE) hospital employees per 1,000 residents
    ◦ Medicare enrollees
    ◦ Total Medicare expenditures per enrollee (Parts A and B) and by setting (SNF, outpatient, physician, home health, hospice, durable medical equipment)
    ◦ Number of surgical dischargers per 1,000 Medicare enrollees.

Statistical Approach

The FDA Form 2830 data contain addresses, including zip codes for each blood establishment. We used a crosswalk to assign an HRR to each zip code. Next, we merged the FDA data with the Dartmouth Atlas market-level data using the HRR. The merged data allowed us to examine how the distribution of blood establishments varied both geographically and by important market characteristics. We have excluded all establishments with non-U.S. addresses ($n = 137$), resulting in 1,019 unique blood establishments in 2016.

We calculated descriptive statistics and cross-tabulations across several measures to characterize the distribution of blood establishments across health care markets. We calculated simple and adjusted correlation coefficients of the number of different types of blood establishments in a market and health care market characteristics (see Chapter Eight). We adjusted for the following market-level measures that might be correlated with blood establishment locations: the number of Medicare enrollees, population, the number of acute-care hospital beds per 1,000 residents, the number of hospital-based registered nurses (RNs), the number of FTE hospital employees per 1,000 residents, the number of surgical discharges per 1,000 Medicare enrollees, and the total number of inpatient discharges.

CHAPTER FOUR

Trends Affecting Blood System Sustainability

As noted in Chapter Two, the blood system is in a period of transition. In particular, some blood centers are facing challenges adapting to evolving market conditions. In this chapter, we focus on understanding how key blood system stakeholders perceive the current blood system challenges in a broader context of change within the entire U.S. health care system. These broader systemic changes include an improved understanding of how to treat patients more effectively by safely using blood less frequently and in smaller quantities, growing demand for health care services because of the ACA coverage expansion, a renewed focus on population health, and evolving incentives for payers and providers due to delivery and payment innovations.

This chapter identifies and describes the most significant external trends affecting the U.S. blood system, taking into account the different perspectives of blood consumers (primarily hospitals); blood suppliers (primarily blood centers); and suppliers of blood-related equipment, goods, and services. To do this, we conducted a political, economic, sociocultural, technological, and legal (PESTL) analysis,[1] drawing on academic and other literature and semi-structured interviews (as described in Chapter Three). We also developed a conceptual framework to illustrate the relationships among the leading trends and to explain their likely effects on different stakeholders in the U.S. blood system.

Methods

PESTL Overview

A PESTL analysis is often used to help organizations understand and characterize the external business environment as part of their strategic planning. To complete the analysis, we gathered a list of trends and then described each one, drawing on mentions and their characterizations in literature and semi-structured interviews. As part of this step, we labeled each trend as "political," "economic," "sociocultural," "technological," or "legal," using the definitions in Figure 4.1. Next, we qualitatively assessed

---

[1] Gemma Massey, "Marketing Environments: The European Airline Industry," Marked by Teachers, 2015.

the importance of each trend, using indicators of salience (described in the following analysis section), and the trend's likely effects on different players in the U.S. blood system, including hospitals, blood suppliers, donors, and the general public.

It should be noted that while the goal of a PESTL analysis is to characterize the external environment, we allowed participants to discuss trends that might directly affect only their business. In such cases, characterizations might only indirectly influence the blood system as a whole. Clearly, what is "external" depends on the perspective of the stakeholder. For this reason, we include trends that could be internal to certain players but external to others.

Semi-structured Interviews and Focus Groups

Our primary data for the PESTL analysis came from semi-structured telephone interviews and focus groups with blood system stakeholders. We interviewed representatives from ten blood centers, eight hospitals, and 11 corporations that supply equipment and services to blood centers and hospitals (hereafter referred to as "suppliers") from February to June 2016 (see Chapter Three for more details on our methodology).

Literature Review

In addition to interviewing blood industry representatives, we examined published literature to identify and describe health care system trends. In our analysis, the literature served as a secondary data source to triangulate findings from the semi-structured interviews and focus groups. We added this additional data source to assess the consistency of information obtained across the different data sources, to verify the accuracy

Figure 4.1
PESTL Domains

Political	Economic	Sociocultural	Technological	Legal
Government stability and initiatives Deregulation Privatization Foreign trade regulation Taxation policy	Business cycles Interest rates Gross national product trends Money supply Credit control Inflation Unemployment Disposable income Competitors' pricing	Population demographics Income distribution Social mobility Lifestyle changes Educational and vocational qualifications Working conditions Attitudes toward work and leisure	Spending on research by government and industry Speed of technology transfer New materials and processes Refinements in equipment, such as robotics and computers Information technology development	Health and safety law Employment regulations Monopoly legislation New restrictions on trade and product standards Restrictions on working hours

SOURCE: Massey, 2015.

of claims made by interview participants, and to help ensure that our analysis of the external environment was rich and comprehensive.

To identify relevant literature, we searched LexisNexis, Google, and PubMed using various combinations of the following keywords: ACA, ACO, blood, blood bank, blood center, blood industry, blood supply, bundled payment, consolidation, coverage expansion, fee schedule change, forecasting, future, health care reform, trends, health care system trends, horizontal integration, marketplace, Medicaid, medical device excise tax (MDET), Medicare, strategic planning, subsidy, and vertical integration. We also limited our searches to literature published from 1999 to 2016, and we excluded documents that did not focus on the U.S health care or blood system.

We extracted text data from a total of 97 documents. These came from the following categories:

- **Media:** print and online newspapers, newswires and press releases, media releases, news transcripts, print and online magazines and journals, print and online newsletters, and web-based publications
- **Legal:** law reviews and journals, U.S. laws, legal news, court cases, and Senate briefings
- **Business publications:** business journals, company websites, company profiles, company filings, online company statements, business school cases, market reports, online briefings, and annual reports
- **Industry:** industry comment letters, industry guidelines, and stakeholder presentations
- **Academic:** peer-reviewed original research articles and commentaries in academic journals

Qualitative Analysis

We used standard qualitative analysis techniques to identify themes and "leading trends" in the interview, focus group, and document data. Following Miles and Huberman,[2] the thematic analysis incorporated both themes and trends identified during the initial literature review (that were included in the interview guides), as well as new unanticipated themes that emerged during the interviews, focus groups, and document review.[3] A hierarchically organized codebook was developed to identify and summarize themes and patterns.[4]

---

[2]   M. B. Miles and A. M. Huberman, *Qualitative Data Analysis: An Expanded Sourcebook*, Thousand Oaks, Calif.: Sage Publications, 1994.

[3]   G. W. Ryan and H. R. Bernard, "Techniques to Identify Themes," *Field Methods*, Vol. 15, No. 1, 2003, pp. 85–109.

[4]   K. MacQueen, E. McLellan, L. Kay, and B. Milstein, "Code Book Development for Team-Based Qualitative Analysis," *CAM Journal*, Vol. 10, 1988, pp. 31–36.

To select the leading health care system trends, we used the following indicators of salience: the number of different reports and interviews that mentioned a particular trend, the amount of space dedicated to a particular trend (i.e., whether entire sections of a report or several minutes of an interview were devoted to it), and consistent conceptualization of a particular trend across a range of stakeholders. To be considered a leading trend, at least ten interview participants representing both stakeholder groups and five or more documents needed to discuss the trend and describe it in a consistent manner. This cutoff was selected following study team review of the distribution of the mentions and occurrences.

We compared leading trends and other themes by respondent type (blood center versus hospital) to assess intergroup differences. Furthermore, all data sources were used to confirm themes identified in interviews or document reviews in order to increase the reliability of our conclusions. MaxQDA Version 10 qualitative research software was used to facilitate data handling, coding, and thematic analyses. Qualitative results are presented as a list of leading trends with illustrative quotes to provide examples of key concepts, followed by secondary trends similarly illustrated.

Results

Leading Trends

Our analysis identified several main trends affecting the blood system and explored the roots of these trends in the broader health care system and other areas.

Reduced Demand for Blood

The most prominent trend identified by both hospitals and blood centers is one we have previously discussed: the declining demand for blood in the past decade. As described by a participant representing a small blood center in the South, "The number one thing affecting us now is decrease in usage." While diverse players consistently cited the trend in the blood system as well as the literature, the trend and its impact were framed differently depending on the stakeholder. For hospital participants, reduced demand for blood was a positive development that was likely to reduce costs and improve patient safety. In contrast, blood centers acknowledged that the decline in demand represents an improvement in patient safety, but centers also considered it a threat to their business and an ongoing source of uncertainty. According to a participant representing a large blood center in the Midwest, "I think I am most worried about how low utilization will go. We don't know. We are not opposed to lower utilization, but we need to rationalize our supply chain against that falling demand."

Documents and interview participants identified several factors contributing to reduced demand: (1) an increase in patient blood management programs; (2) a continued trend toward less-invasive surgeries; (3) pharmacologic agents, such as erythropoietin or tranexamic acid, that eliminate the need for transfusion in some situations; (4)

expansion of services provided by clinics, which are less likely to stock and use blood; and (5) revised transfusion guidelines from professional societies (e.g., lower hemoglobin and platelet count thresholds) that reduce the number of patient transfusions.[5] Furthermore, all data sources predicted that this trend would continue, with one source suggesting that blood utilization in the United States is still higher than it should be and another source from a trauma center suggesting that usage was expected to continue to decline.[6]

In contrast with national statistics from the 2011 NBCUS, in which 30 percent of hospitals in the U.S. reported having a patient blood management program, most hospitals participating in our interviews had a patient blood management program that has reduced blood use by up to 10 percent since its implementation. As more U.S. hospitals introduce patient blood management programs, we can expect similar declines in blood use. Programs typically featured educational components geared toward helping providers make better decisions, clinical decision support tools to limit the number of units ordered, and feedback to individual physicians about their transfusion practices. For example, one representative from a trauma center noted that many providers were still using older thresholds of hemoglobin concentrations of 8 to 9 g/dL, whereas evidence suggests that a transfusion threshold of 7 g/dL is safer for patients;[7] the center has since pushed to increase awareness of this evidence among providers. The center also made a change in the electronic health ordering system that required physicians to order one unit of blood at a time.

Participants generally agreed that demand for blood would continue to decline, with several mentioning that an aging population could at some point mitigate the downward trend. The effect of an aging population, however, is not straightforward, as the donor base tends to be older on average,[8] but older individuals also tend to need more health services, including transfusions.

Shrinking Profits for Blood Centers and Their Suppliers

Every participating blood center and many of their suppliers mentioned the trend of shrinking profit margins for blood centers, and several blood centers commented that the payment they receive from hospitals for blood does not adequately cover their production costs. One supplier suggested that over half of the existing blood centers are losing money on a per-unit basis. Although this was a major concern for most blood

---

[5]   Negin, 2015; Marks, Epstein, and Borio, 2016; Nielsen and Nielsen, 2016; McCullough, McCullough, and Riley, 2016.

[6]   Nielsen and Nielsen, 2016.

[7]   J. P. AuBuchon, K. Puca, S. Saxena, I. Shulman, and J. Waters, *Getting Started in Patient Blood Management*, Bethesda, Md.: American Association of Blood Banks, 2011.

[8]   Shimian Zou, Fatemeh Musavi, Edward P. Notari, Chyang T. Fang, and ARCNET Research Group., "Changing Age Distribution of the Blood Donor Population in the United States," *Transfusion*, Vol. 48, No. 2, 2008, pp. 251–257.

centers in our sample, one manager of a large blood center stated that this trend primarily affects centers focused only on collecting and processing blood, whereas the manager's organization had been less affected because it was much more diversified. Hospital representatives also recognized the trend, although they, unlike their blood center counterparts, rarely expressed dissatisfaction with the price for blood or their contracts with blood suppliers. However, one manager from a hospital GPO stated that some blood centers have been regional monopolies for some time and that competition is a positive development that will allow blood center prices to fall. Online blood brokers, such as Bloodbuy, also recognize this trend as a business opportunity, potentially motivating organizations to move more of their blood sales and purchases to online platforms.

Numerous blood center representatives noted that their profit margins were shrinking because hospitals had growing power in contract negotiations and were increasingly concerned about containing costs. As explained by a representative from a small blood center, "The terms are changing rapidly. It used to be that blood prices were set by the center. Today, pricing is driven by requests for proposals [RFPs] or hospitals are essentially dictating price. Generally, they inform us what they are willing to pay, and we have to accept that, or they will find someone else who will." Other blood centers mentioned an inability to increase prices for newer tests or increases in other costs.

Blood center representatives listed a variety of potential downstream effects of shrinking profit margins, including worsening service (e.g., less frequent restocking, emergency deliveries, and education programs), less investment in innovation, and blood shortages. Similarly, their suppliers unanimously emphasized the downstream negative effects on innovation. One supplier of blood collection and processing equipment stated that centers were trying to pass on cost declines to suppliers, but profit margins for suppliers were often so low that it was not worthwhile for them to manufacture certain low-margin products and equipment for blood centers.

Although declining profit margins were a common theme in blood center interviews, it is worth noting that a more-thorough empirical analysis would be needed to better understand the accounting underlying these concerns. For example, it could be that the marginal cost of producing one additional unit of blood is lower than the market price hospitals pay; however, once additional fixed costs are factored in, profit margins become negative. The marginal cost reflects the incremental additional cost of selling one additional unit and, therefore, ignores fixed costs (it assumes that they are "sunk"). The policy implications are different in the case where the marginal cost is greater than the market price of blood and in the case where the marginal cost is less than the market price, which indicates loss on each additional unit sold. In the former case, we would want to understand how fixed costs could be changed (in the longer run), whereas in the latter case, both fixed and variable costs are too high relative to the market price, suggesting that blood centers would exit the market if the market price, fixed costs, or variable costs do not change.

Shrinking Donor Pool

Hospital and blood center participants, as well as multiple documents, identified the problem of the shrinking supply of donors and expressed concern about how this trend will adversely affect all stakeholders in the blood industry.[9] Interview participants and documents directly noted a reduction (or anticipated reduction) in donations caused by a variety of trends, including (1) aging donors, (2) increasing exclusion criteria and deferrals, and (3) reduced investment in donor recruitment by the blood centers.

One study noted, "The age cohort with the highest donation rate is aging out of eligibility."[10] One small blood center noted that the majority of their committed donors were older than age 55. Travel deferrals and other exclusion criteria are also causing challenges, as the older donor base tends to include individuals who are more likely to travel or have medical deferrals. In addition, as the number of emerging pathogens continues to increase, there might be even more deferrals.[11]

Although several articles and blood center representatives noted that the shrinking donor pool might require blood centers to increase expenditures on donor recruitment in the future to maintain an adequate supply, one hospital representative from a large mid-Atlantic hospital commented that some of the donor supply issues might be attributed to less-intensive outreach by blood centers as a result of shrinking profit margins.[12]

Understanding the influence of the shrinking donor pool is complicated, as we might expect a decline in the supply of blood to offset the already documented decline in the demand for blood. Although there were fewer individuals presenting to donate in 2011 versus 2008 (17.9 million versus 19.3 million), the percentage of deferrals and

[9] David Green, "Blood Systems' Perspective on State of the Current Blood System," Washington, D.C.: Blood Systems Inc., November 9, 2015; Joshua L. Kwan, "Blood Banks Desperate Runaway Costs: Need Outpaces Donations," San Jose Mercury News, December 6, 1999; Heather Stauffer, "Blood Donors Always Needed; Health Care Local Centers See Drop in Donations Mitigating Factor What They're Trying," LNP, December 11, 2015; Robert Trigaux, "Three-Way Blood Bank Merger in Florida Yields a Behemoth," Tampa Bay Times, January 21, 2012a; Fred V. Plapp, "Future of Transfusion Medicine & Blood Banking," Heart of America Association of Blood Banks, 2013; W. Riley, M. Schwei, and J. McCullough, "The United States' Potential Blood Donor Pool: Estimating the Prevalence of Donor-Exclusion Factors on the Pool of Potential Donors," Transfusion, Vol. 47, 2007, pp. 1180–1188.

[10] Zou et al., 2008.

[11] Harvey J. Alter, Susan L. Stramer, and Roger Y. Dodd, "Emerging Infectious Diseases That Threaten the Blood Supply," Seminars in Hematology, Vol. 44, No. 1, 2007, pp. 32–41; R. Y. Dodd, "Emerging Pathogens and Their Implications for the Blood Supply and Transfusion Transmitted Infections," British Journal of Haematology, Vol. 159, No. 2, 2007, pp. 135–142.

[12] Eric Pera, "Local Blood Bank to Take Part in Nationwide Test; the Test Will Safeguard Against HIV, Hepatitis C," The Ledger, April 1, 1999; Green, 2015; Nielsen and Nielsen, 2016.

the total U.S. population both increased over that period.[13] At the same time, the number of units rejected in testing actually declined from 2008 to 2011. Thus, the extent to which a shrinking donor pool is posing challenges is unclear, particularly in light of improvements in screening and test sensitivity and increases in the population that might offset declines from deferrals or an aging donor population. However, in the event of an emergency, when the system typically relies on the donor pool to provide extra blood, the shrinking pool could be problematic.

Hospital Consolidation

Hospital consolidation was a common theme in interviews with blood centers and was reflected in recent literature.[14] From the perspective of the blood centers, the role of hospital consolidation in the industry is twofold. First, it gives hospitals more purchasing power in contract negotiations and, as such, is further eroding blood center profits. Second, it has increased hospital demand for products and services from larger suppliers of blood and related services with broader geographic and product scope. One large blood center representative noted that blood prices have dropped significantly in the wake of hospital consolidations. We discuss this further in Chapter Eight using the FDA Form 2830 data merged with market-level data; we cannot explicitly examine causal effects of hospital consolidation, but we examine associations between the number of blood centers in a given market and hospital market concentration.

Some interviewees have suggested that hospital consolidation is putting pressure on blood centers to consolidate because consolidated hospitals or systems usually want a single supplier. Although fewer but larger blood centers might strengthen their market position and allow them to bid on large contracts that require supplying blood to multiple hospitals within a system, it is worth noting that many hospitals

---

[13]   HHS, 2011a; HHS, 2011b.

[14]   John D. Oravecz, "Central Blood Bank Parent in Merger Talks with Florida System," *TRIB LIVE*, July 28, 2014; Peter J. Castagna Jr. and Pascal George, "Lehigh Valley and Central New Jersey Blood Centers Announce Intent to Merge Operations," Bethlehem, Pa.: Miller-Keystone Blood Center, November 5, 2014; Green, 2015; Nielsen and Nielsen, 2016; Chris Hrouda, "The American Red Cross," presentation to the HHS Advisory Committee on Blood and Tissue Safety and Availability, Washington, D.C., 2015; Tammie Smith, "A Transfusion of Vision," *Richmond Times Dispatch*, October 29, 2012; "Blood Transfusion Sale Set to Give Novartis a £1Bn Shot in the Arm," *City A.M. Reporter*, November 12, 2013; Bill Toland, "To Cut Costs, More Blood Banks Merge; Officials Cite Need for New Model," *Pittsburgh Post-Gazette*, July 31, 2014; "Blood Centers Announce Merger Intent," *Thomasville Times-Enterprise*, July 25, 2014; India Pharma News, "Global RFID Blood Monitoring Systems Market Is Expected to Reach USD 40.9 Million in 2012: Transparency Market Research," Contify.com, January 11, 2014; TBNweekly.com, "OneBlood Considers Blood Bank Merger," July 30, 2014; National Association of Social Workers, "Blood Banks Serving Polk County to Merge," *The Ledger*, 2015; Trigaux, 2012a; Robert Trigaux, "After This Mega-Deal, Call Them Big Blood," *Tampa Bay Times*, January 22, 2012b; OneBlood and the Institute for Transfusion Medicine, "Blood Centers Announce Intent to Merge," LifeSource, July 25, 2014; and Kenneth Kaufman, "Fast and Furious Blood Industry Decline Sends a Message to the Healthcare Industry," white paper, 2014.

noted having both primary and secondary suppliers. A truly consolidated blood center market might make it difficult for hospitals to have multiple suppliers.[15]

Blood Center Alliances and Consolidation

Multiple blood center and hospital representatives discussed the trend of blood center consolidation, but stakeholders had diverse perspectives on the issue. Several blood centers and hospitals believed that consolidation would reduce excess capacity in the industry and improve service. In particular, mergers and acquisitions could help to solve the excess capacity of suppliers in the industry (specifically, by removing unnecessary fixed costs). On the other hand, one hospital and a handful of blood centers expressed concerns about consolidation leading to reductions in services offered by blood centers to hospital customers, such as transfusion medicine consultations, decline in resources and expertise to support a local donor base, and reduced availability of specialized blood products. Despite these responses, we note that these services and products could still be offered by more consolidated blood centers.

Historically, U.S. blood centers performed most of the blood tests required to screen for diseases and to identify blood type, antigens, and more. More recently, many U.S. blood centers, including those operated by DoD, have either outsourced testing services or consolidated in-house blood testing services, in part to save money by increasing the volume of testing, which reduces the cost per unit.

Secondary Trends

Workforce Shortages

Personnel shortages were a recurring concern among blood centers and hospitals. In particular, finding individuals with the technical (particularly laboratory) expertise is a challenge for the industry. Others have noted the effects of aging blood center leadership. Without a sufficiently large cadre of young blood center managers rising in the ranks, some blood center managers might look to mergers as a solution to succession problems.

Evolving Health Information Technology Environment

A handful of participants observed that health IT is playing an increasingly important role in the blood industry. In many respects, the industry relies on a relatively antiquated system for many tasks that could be automated or streamlined with better-integrated IT platforms. For example, the need for blood centers to call hospitals daily to check stock levels could be reduced if information technology systems across hospitals and blood centers were better connected.

---

[15] Oravecz, 2014; Negin, 2015; Toland, 2014; Chris Morris and Shawn Berry, "Nebraska Blood Service a Model for Success," *The Telegraph-Journal (New Brunswick)*, November 26, 2011; National Association of Social Workers, "Blood Banks Serving Polk County to Merge," *The Ledger*, 2015.

Hospitals were often interested in health IT in the context of supporting efforts to decrease blood use through patient blood management programs, that, for example, provide real-time clinical decision support tools in the electronic health record interface to prevent overuse of blood transfusions.

Declining R&D Investments, Lack of Innovation

R&D investment in the blood system can play an important part in generating innovation and improving product quality, safety, and cost-efficiency. Multiple interview participants commented that blood centers and other industry players did not have the money to invest in R&D because of declining profit margins and FDA hurdles; blood centers and suppliers mentioned this issue more frequently than did their hospital counterparts.

Some managers of U.S. blood centers expressed concerns about declining levels of R&D investment, while others explained why their R&D budgets were more secure. One vice president of a blood center with a national presence stated that since 2007 his

> R&D budget has shrunk every year … the most massive cuts have come in the last five or six years. Our budget has been cut more than 50% since its peak … blood centers can no longer afford to support doing research and we can't charge for research nor make enough margin to make up for it.

However, some blood centers focused on R&D reported relying on more diversified sources of revenue, including foundations with patent revenues or philanthropic donors, while others said that they relied on NIH grants. Furthermore, interview participants identified additional barriers to innovation, including FDA, the DRG system of reimbursement, and, most importantly, the unwillingness of hospitals to pay for unmandated innovations that add to costs.

FDA has been occasionally criticized for taking too long to respond to new technology applications, which some blood centers claimed increases the cost of R&D investment. However, others have noted that FDA can play an important role in ushering in new R&D investment by imposing requirements (and thereby creating demand) for additional tests or PRTs. However, because of the way hospitals are reimbursed (see Chapter Five), some have argued that they have little incentive to pay for some of these innovations, as it typically takes two to three years before increased costs are reflected in DRG reimbursement rates.

Several participants explained that because hospitals are extremely cost-conscious, they are reluctant to pay for innovations, such as new safety measures, unless they are explicitly required. As explained by a representative from a large hospital in the Midwest,

> My concern relates more to safety. I would like to see additional use of pathogen inactivation. . . . Cost is holding blood centers back from adding safety measures.

If adding pathogen inactivation to platelets and plasma, you're adding $60 to $70 per unit; the hospital is not going to pay for that.

The representative from a large Mid-Atlantic hospital noted,

I think there are innovations that are being developed that will affect patient safety. But I worry if they will be affordable in the current environment. I like pathogen inactivation systems that are potentially coming to market, but these will require added costs because of the more expensive technology. These things may be slow to be adopted by hospitals and blood centers because they are not perceived as affordable. Better blood therapies for patients may cost more and can have benefits, but there is inhibited progress with this in [the] current environment.

Suppliers voiced similar concerns. A blood testing device manufacturer stated,

Regulatory requirements and costs of compliance make it very hard to invest in new technologies or even update current ones unless there is a very large market potential. These requirements erect barriers to entry for smaller players, but also can hurt larger players as well who may not find enough return on investment after dealing with regulatory burdens.

More Frequent Public Health Emergencies

There is evidence that public health emergencies, including emerging infectious diseases, will grow in frequency in the coming years because of such factors as climate change, urbanization, population growth, and environmental degradation.[16] Several blood suppliers and hospitals expressed concern that, although the U.S. blood system works during routine times, it is very vulnerable to emerging threats, such as the Zika virus, and other public health disasters. A representative from a large trauma center explained, "I worry about extraordinary circumstance/disaster. For the middle of the road, the system works."

Stakeholders pointed out that such threats could produce surges in demand for blood that could not be met and could also disrupt the supply. As described by a representative from a large hospital, "Shortages can be a big problem during blizzards. With the recent blizzard [the 2015 blizzard in the Northeast], the [local] platelet supply was not what it needed to be. This is more of an issue of donors. Donors aren't going to go out and donate when there is a blizzard." A representative from a large blood center with a national presence noted that he was increasingly fielding questions from hospi-

---

[16] Sophie Adams, Florent Baarsch, Alberte Bondeau, Dim Coumou, Reik Donner, Katja Frieler, Bill Hare, Arathy Menon, Mahe Perette, Franziska Piontek, Kira Rehfeld, Alexander Robinson, Marcia Rocha, Joeri Rogelj, Jakob Runge, Michiel Schaeffer, Jacob Schewe, Carl-Friedrich Schleussner, Susanne Schwan, Olivia Serdeczny, Anastasia Svirejeva-Hopkins, Marion Vieweg, Lila Warszawski, and World Bank, *Turn Down the Heat: Climate Extremes, Regional Impacts, and the Case for Resilience*, Washington, D.C., World Bank, 2013, pp. 1–255.

tals about the center's ability and resources (e.g., communications systems) to "handle huge surges in demand in cases of mass casualty incidents."

Zika was frequently mentioned, with two interview participants expressing concern that all the blood collected in certain cities or states would have to be discarded in certain circumstances. A representative from a medium-sized blood center in the South posed the question, "If we shut down blood centers in Miami and Houston and other major cities [as a result of Zika], what is the country's ability for other places/cities to take up the slack?"

Currently, the U.S. blood system seems to respond to these types of emergencies by relying on secondary markets and the government for assistance. For example, with declines in transportation costs over time, it is not uncommon for hospitals and blood centers to purchase blood from blood centers that are net exporters (e.g., areas with a large donor base and lower demand for blood) to areas of the country where demand exceeds supply (e.g., coastal areas or areas with large cancer treatment centers). In the case of weather-related emergencies, movement of blood from one part of the country to another can offset declines in donations. Such solutions, however, are only feasible to the extent that distributors can actually reach hospitals in affected areas. It might be difficult to get shipments to hospitals where roads were covered by snow or destroyed by an earthquake, for example. In such cases involving high intensity short-term emergencies, existing government infrastructure may be of little help. However, in the case of slower-moving emergencies, such as that caused by the spread of the Zika virus, the HHS Secretary's Operations Center (SOC) can step in to facilitate shipment of blood to affected areas, as it did with Puerto Rico in early 2016.

New Contracting Approaches

Some blood centers mentioned increasing pressures from greater use of a competitive bidding process in which hospitals issue requests for proposals to which all blood centers can respond, improvements in shipping that allow distant blood centers to compete with local ones, and willingness or ability of some of the larger or more-diversified blood centers to lose money to keep prices low. According to a representative from a small blood center,

> One of the newest phenomena over the past 3–4 years is the use of consultants and brokers where hospitals hire someone to run an RFP process for them. This used to be common in the health insurance market, not so in the blood bank market . . . . The RFP process is quite new in blood banks. This has dramatically reduced prices. You are forcing competition to where there was none.

However, this trend might not be representative of all acquisition approaches of hospitals. According to a GPO manager, hospital blood consumers have been hurt in the past by "regional and local monopolies" that blood centers controlled, and, from her perspective, the introduction of RFPs has improved competition. Earlier studies suggested significant geographic variation in the prices that blood centers charged, which might be caused by both differences in underlying costs of production (e.g., greater regulatory costs in California) and differences in regional demand.[17] Blood centers that collect more blood than is needed locally (net exporters) can sell surplus blood to other centers. Bloodbuy, the NBE, or other exchange platforms facilitate these types of transactions. Although transaction-level data are not publicly available, net exporter blood centers likely charge different prices in these exchanges than they charge local hospitals. With large players, such as ARC, controlling large parts of the market, there may be other effects on prices. Independent blood bankers have suggested that ARC, diversified both geographically and across product lines, can afford to sell blood at lower-than-market prices. For example, ARC admitted to subsidizing prices in parts of California where production costs were greater than average.[18]

Thus, these dynamics make it difficult to know exactly what the effects of the market structure are on prices. There are likely downward pressures on prices aside from the declines in the demand for blood, but they are likely driven by the market structures of both blood centers and hospitals.

Additional Trends
Affordable Care Act

The ACA was mentioned quickly or in passing by several interview participants and across multiple documents; however, the effects of the ACA on the blood industry were seldom conceptualized in the same way.[19] The ACA could be invoked as (1) a force likely to increase demand for blood (i.e., as new patients gain insurance and demand more procedures that require blood transfusions), (2) the impetus for hospital consolidation and other changes to the organization of the health care system, (3) the reason hospitals are becoming more cost-conscious in contracting negotiations and demanding lower prices for blood, or (4) the reason hospitals are working to reduce blood utilization (i.e., because of pay for value and the need to provide high-quality care at lower costs).[20] Overall, there is no uniform agreement on whether the ACA will materially affect the blood system and, if so, in which way.

Medical Device Excise Tax

The MDET is a 2.3-percent federal tax on medical devices that went into effect in 2013 as a result of the implementation of the ACA. Although no interview participants

---

[17] Goodman et al., 2003.

[18] Goodman et al., 2003.

[19] Plapp, 2013; TBNWeekly.com, 2014; Toland, 2014; Kenneth Kaufman, "Blood Banks Unite to Better Serve Coachella Valley," *The Desert Sun*, May 17, 2012; Fred Hiers, "OneBlood Seeks Partner, a Sign of the Times," *Ocala Star-Banner*, 2014; Bloodbuy, "For Hospitals," undated; Biologics Direct, "Nation's Blood Distribution Undergoes Major Changes," Alex Garcia and Charles Rouault, March 16, 2015.

[20] Morris and Berry, 2011; Bloodbuy, undated.

mentioned this tax, a small number of documents identified the MDET as a concerning trend for blood suppliers.[21] The lack of attention to the MDET by interview participants can be attributed to a two-year moratorium on the MDET that went into effect on January 1, 2016, and continues through December 31, 2017, during which time the application of the MDET to the sale of a taxable medical device by the manufacturer, producer, or importer is prohibited.[22] However, select documents revealed that blood bank officials were concerned that device manufacturers would pass the cost along to them if the MDET were to be implemented.[23] The MDET was consistently conceptualized as a threat to blood center profitability because it conceivably will increase blood center operating costs.

Limitations

There are various limitations to our analysis of external factors affecting the U.S. blood system. First, although the participating eight hospitals, eight suppliers, and nine blood centers were selected to represent the diversity of these entities in the blood system (e.g., with respect to geography, size), our sample was essentially a convenience sample. Second, by focusing our primary data collection efforts on hospitals, blood centers, and suppliers for this chapter, we did not obtain the perspectives of all the stakeholders in the U.S. blood system. This focus on three existing groups of stakeholders might also overemphasize the perspectives of organizations with a vested interest in maintaining the status quo. In other words, this chapter might not sufficiently emphasize outside perspectives from organizations wishing to disrupt the status quo in ways that might further improve the blood system. However, although our interviews were limited to blood centers, suppliers, and hospitals, our literature review had no such restrictions and, as such, helped to address these limitations.

---

[21]   Smith, 2012; Hologic Inc., "FDA Expands Emergency Use Authorization for Hologic's Aptima Zika Virus Assay to Include Use with Urine Samples," press release, September 8, 2016; Thomas Zadvyas, "Sense of the Markets: Clarity Drives Medtech Deals," *Daily Deal/The Deal*, May 10, 2010; J. K. Wall, "Outlook Gloomy for Medical Device Investments," *Indianapolis Business Journal*, November 2012; Steve Adams, "Health Reform to Leave Its Mark; Consumers, Businesses, Biotech May Benefit in Massachusetts," *The Patriot Ledger*, March 27, 2010; ABC, "America's Blood Centers Opposes Healthcare Reform Legislation that Imposes Fee or Tax on Medical Devices Sold to Blood Centers," Washington, D.C.: ABC, 2009.

[22]   Dent, 2015; Internal Revenue Service, 2016.

[23]   Smith, 2012; Adams, 2010; ABC, 2009.

Conclusions

We identified five leading trends and seven more minor (secondary and additional) trends that our key stakeholders perceived as affecting or having the potential to affect the U.S. blood system. The majority of the trends were economic or technological, with far fewer sociocultural, legal, and political trends in the external environment. Hospital participants had far fewer concerns than blood centers about the future of the U.S. blood system or their role in it. Their silence on many of these trends is suggestive evidence that hospitals are faring relatively well in this changing system. On the other hand, blood centers and their suppliers were a more-vocal group and were more directly threatened by recent trends.

Stakeholders and previous scientific literature identified trends at various levels, including those upstream and downstream. In addition, they did not always acknowledge the interrelatedness of select trends. To help explain the relationships among the trends identified, we created a conceptual framework of the external environment in which the blood system is operating (Figure 4.2). A leading trend (both driving and driven by other trends) is the declining profits of blood centers; thus, it is in the center of the figure. Lower profit margins are a result of several trends in the blood industry, including reduced demand for blood, hospital consolidation (which has increased the purchasing power of hospitals), and a shrinking donor base (which will increase costs associated with donor recruitment). Whereas hospital consolidation is in part driven by

Figure 4.2
Relationships Among Trends Affecting the Blood Industry

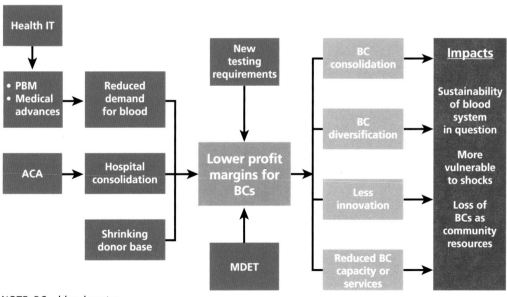

NOTE: BC = blood center.

RAND *RR1575-4.2*

the implementation of the ACA, the reduced demand for blood is driven by changes in clinical practice, including new surgical techniques and patient blood management programs. Health IT supports and facilitates blood conservation strategies, such as patient blood management. For example, clinical decision support can help ensure that physicians are ordering blood in accordance with guidelines.

As a result of declining profits, blood centers are consolidating or joining networks and partnerships in an effort to increase efficiency and competitiveness. To some extent, they are also trying to remove excess capacity from the industry (e.g., cutting staff) and eliminating uncompensated services, such as educational programs. In select cases, they have also reduced investment in innovation. Lower profit margins have also led some blood centers to diversify and enter new areas beyond the provision of blood, such as iron supplement injections, organ testing services, or hospital consulting services. At the same time, other blood centers have shed some of their functions to cut costs, such as outsourcing blood testing to specialized organizations or cutting back on education or technical consultation services to hospitals.

All of these trends together have certain long-term implications for the U.S. blood industry. As a result of the downstream effects of lower profit margins for blood centers, the U.S. blood system may be more vulnerable to demand and supply side shocks, and blood centers may have less of a community presence, which can affect their responsiveness to local needs and customer service, as well as their ability to recruit donors. However, there are several potential positive effects from the hospital and societal perspective, including lower prices for blood and increased patient safety because of fewer unnecessary blood transfusions.

Trends affecting the broader U.S. health system will continue to influence and transform the blood system. Trends in the external environment interact with and affect the blood sector in a multitude of ways, but our analysis indicates that the leading trends include

- declining demand for blood
- shrinking profits for blood centers
- a shrinking pool of active donors
- hospital consolidation
- an increase in blood center alliances and mergers.

In the following chapters, we further examine the policy implications of these trends, including how they might affect the sustainability and resilience of the U.S. blood system and how adopting new payment methods and selected best practices from other countries' blood systems might help to further strengthen the U.S. blood system.

CHAPTER FIVE

Payment for Blood and Health Care Services Involving Blood

Introduction

As described in Chapter Four, several of the key trends related to blood system sustainability are economic, including declining demand for blood and shrinking blood center profit margins. This chapter examines the economics of the U.S blood system in more detail, with an emphasis on current policies for paying for blood and blood-related health care services, potential alternative policies, and the potential of alternative policies to improve sustainability.

There are two key economic relationships at the core of the U.S. blood system: the relationship between hospitals and blood suppliers and the relationship between hospitals and health care payers (see Figure 5.1). In the first relationship, hospitals pay blood centers for products and services, usually on a per-unit basis and under a consignment model. These contractual arrangements often outline specific service requirements (such as delivery frequency), payment mechanisms (such as payment on delivery versus consignment), and payment rates. The requirements and rates set in these agreements are key determinants of the financial well-being and sustainability of blood centers.

Figure 5.1
Payment and Product Flow

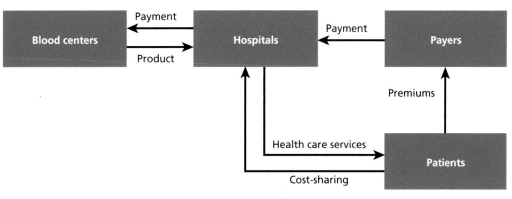

RAND *RR1575-5.1*

The second relationship involves payments from public and private health care payers to hospitals and other providers for health care services involving blood, including surgeries, oncology treatment, and childbirth services. Payment rates and arrangements vary significantly by payer, geography, and type of service. Although payers have historically compensated providers on a fee-for-service basis, newer payment models aim to reduce unnecessary or low-value care through single payments covering entire episodes of care. This is particularly true for inpatient care, where most payers pay predetermined rates per hospital stay depending on a diagnosis. Regardless of whether a specific payment arrangement is fee-for-service or episode-based, hospitals often can increase their margins, at least in the short term, by decreasing the production costs involved in delivering health care services, including the costs associated with purchasing blood. This is one contributing factor to downward pressure on blood prices.

In the inpatient setting—where the majority of blood is used[1]—there are no immediate links between payments received by hospitals and payments flowing from hospitals to blood centers. In Medicare, which accounted for 39 percent and 46 percent of inpatient hospital stays and costs in 2013, respectively,[2] hospitals receive the same predetermined payment per inpatient stay regardless of whether or how much blood is used. And, if blood is used, hospitals pay blood centers at negotiated prices that do not vary with the payments they receive for the stay. The disconnect between payments to hospitals and payments from hospitals to suppliers applies to some drugs, medical devices, equipment, and other inputs into hospital care, in addition to blood. The motivation for this kind of payment arrangement in the U.S. health care system is to put the onus on hospitals to be cost-conscious providers of care.

This chapter describes the status quo for payment relationships, describes a framework to categorize policy changes from the status quo, and provides estimates of the effects of a set of potential policies on stakeholders. It is important to note that the disconnect between payments to hospitals and payments to blood centers results in important limitations of some policy approaches that aim to improve the financial situation of blood centers. For example, policies increasing payments to hospitals with the aim of revenue "spilling over" to blood centers would not necessarily work because hospitals have an incentive to retain as large a margin as possible.

Summary of Methods

Our description of current payment arrangements and challenges draws from interviews of blood center and hospital stakeholders, blood center focus groups, and ad hoc

---

[1]   Chung et al, 2016.

[2]   Celeste Torio and Brian Moore, "National Inpatient Hospital Costs: The Most Expensive Conditions by Payer, 2013," Statistical Brief No. 204, Agency for Healthcare Research and Quality, May 2016.

conversations with stakeholders. Chapter Three describes in detail our methods for this primary data collection. For the results described in this chapter, we synthesized payment-related information by theme.

We used NBCUS data to describe current payments from hospitals to blood centers. We also used CMS data to describe current payments to hospitals for services involving blood. Chapter Two contains details on these data sources and our approach to linking data.

Status Quo Payment Arrangements

Payments to Blood Centers

Hospitals negotiate agreements with blood centers that usually specify levels of supply and services provided by the blood center in exchange for per-unit payments from the hospital. The most-common type of agreement is a consignment model in which a blood center delivers blood to a hospital, but the hospital pays only for the units of blood used. As a result, blood centers bear the risk for outdated units. To minimize this risk, centers attempt to transport blood between hospitals to where it is most likely to be used. Under a second model, the payment-upon-delivery model, a hospital pays for and owns units when they are delivered. In either case, blood centers do not have any incentive to limit use in terms of units transfused (in fact, they are financially better off when use is higher), while hospitals directly reduce their expenditures and improve margins by using less blood (assuming a fixed payment for the inpatient stay).

Blood center interviewees reported that other payment models—such as per-patient models where the hospitals pay blood centers a fixed rate per inpatient discharge or patient-day regardless of blood use—are only rarely used. Per-patient payment could lead to different incentives for blood centers and hospitals compared with per-unit consignment payment. Specifically, hospitals would not have the incentive to limit utilization because they pay a single per-patient price regardless of the number of units transfused, while blood centers paid on a per-patient basis could have a more-predictable revenue stream.

Regardless of the choice of primary payment agreement—either per-unit consignment, payment on delivery, capitation, or another model—secondary agreements are common to ensure the availability of blood in the event of local, temporary shortages and of rare blood products. These arrangements can either flow through the hospital's primary blood supplier (e.g., in which the primary blood center acquires a necessary product from another blood center and then bills the hospital at the usual rate, at a different rate, or with an acquisition fee) or through a secondary arrangement with a large blood supplier like ARC. Interview participants reported that it is common for blood purchased by hospitals through these secondary arrangements to be paid for on a per-unit basis but without consignment—that is, the hospital purchases and owns the product on delivery.

The prices paid by hospitals for blood have been generally stable over time in nominal terms. The average price paid from hospitals to blood centers for a unit of leuko-reduced RBCs increased in nominal terms from $211.50 in 2006 to $225.74 in 2013, with a 5-percent increase from 2006 to 2008 and virtually no change in price from 2008 to 2013.[3] Over the same time period, the hospital producer price index— a measure of the change in cost for inputs into hospital care maintained by the U.S. Bureau of Labor Statistics[4]—increased by 21 percent, suggesting that the price that hospitals pay for blood has increased more slowly than the prices they pay for other inputs in aggregate. After adjusting for inflation, the price for a unit of leuko-reduced RBCs fell by 11 percent from 2008 to 2013 (in constant 2013 dollars; see Figure 5.2). As described next, decreasing prices paid for blood translate in the short term to savings for hospitals; in the long term, they result in savings to Medicare and other health care payers and, ultimately, to taxpayers and beneficiaries paying premiums for insurance coverage.

Payments to Hospitals

Hospitals receive payments from health insurers and individuals (in the case of cost-sharing) in exchange for health care services. The most common approach used by insurers to pay hospitals depends on whether the care is provided in the inpatient setting—that is, when the patient is admitted to the hospital—or an ambulatory setting—for example, in a hospital outpatient department (HOPD) or emergency department. Payments for hospital and other health care services across the U.S. health care system tend to follow the lead of Medicare, the largest single payer for health care in the United States, run by CMS. As a result, we describe Medicare's general approach to payment in the inpatient and ambulatory settings while detailing notable trends and innovation in payment within CMS and among other public and private payers in a separate section.

Facility Payments for Care Delivered in the Inpatient Setting

Medicare payment for inpatient care is typically a single, diagnosis-specific payment covering an entire hospital stay, regardless of length of stay or the specific services delivered to the patient during the stay. Medicare and many other payers use a DRG system to classify inpatient hospital stays into categories based on principal diagnosis, complications and comorbidities, and surgical procedures, each of which is assigned a payment rate ahead of time. Because Medicare's payment for inpatient care is a fixed

---

3   Analyses based on survey results from three consecutive NBCUS reports: HHS, 2011a; HHS, 2011b; Chung et al., 2016.

4   Bureau of Labor Statistics, "Hospital Producer Price Index," 2016.

Figure 5.2
Average Hospital Payments per Unit, by Product, 2006 to 2013

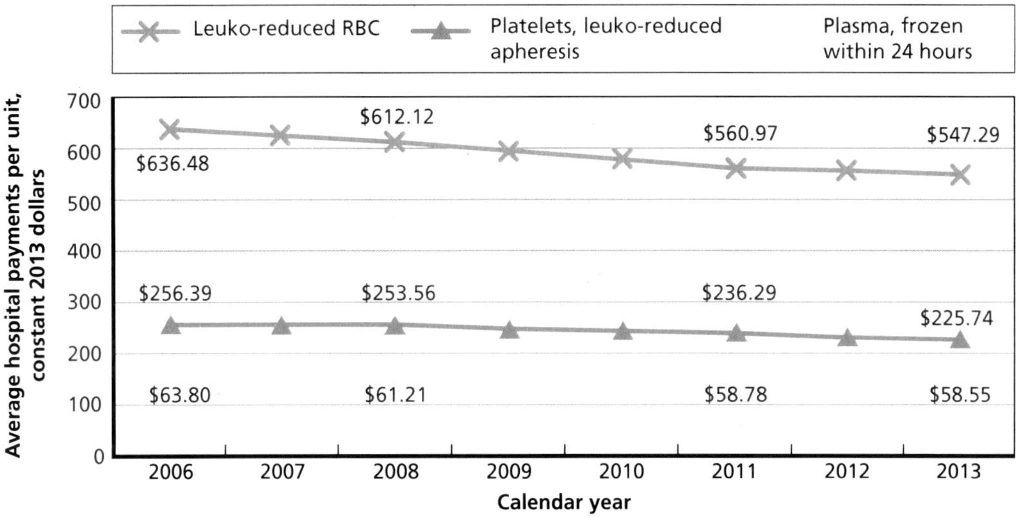

SOURCE: RAND analysis of estimates from the 2009 NBCUS report; 2011 NBCUS report; and 2013 NBCUS report (HHS, 2011a; HHS, 2011b; HHS, 2013). Prices are linearly interpolated for 2007, 2009, 2010, and 2012, as there were no NBCUS estimates for these years. Inflation adjustment is from the Bureau of Labor Statistics 2016 Hospital Producer Price Index.
RAND *RR1575-5.2*

amount per stay, subject to adjustments for outliers, teaching hospitals, and other factors, hospitals face financial incentives to provide services and use inputs into care—including labor, supplies, drugs, and units of blood for transfusions—only when necessary because they are not paid at higher rates if they transfuse additional units.

In 2007, Medicare adopted Medicare severity-adjusted DRGs (MS-DRGs), a set of DRGs specific to resource use and disease severity in Medicare beneficiaries. Medicare reports aggregate data for charges per MS-DRG—that is, the amount billed by hospitals—and hospital costs annually as part of its rulemaking process.[5] Tables 5.1 through 5.3 report top MS-DRGs by (1) aggregate national total charges, (2) aggregate national blood charges, and (3) share of charges that are associated with blood. Blood charges account for 0.1 percent to 2.1 percent of total charges for the top ten MS-DRGs by volume (Table 5.1). Across all MS-DRGs, hospitals reported $4.60 billion in Medicare charges associated with blood out of $442.5 billion in total Medicare charges. The MS-DRGs associated with the highest aggregate blood charges include a mix of MS-DRGs with large total charges overall (e.g., septicemia or severe sepsis, MS-DRG 871, with 1.0 percent of total charges associated with blood), as well as less

---

5   CMS, "CMS-1632-F and IFC, CMS-1632-CN2 and Changes Due to the Consolidated Appropriations Act of 2016: Final Rule, Correction Notice and the Consolidated Appropriations Act of 2016," Baltimore, Md., 2016a.

Table 5.1
Top MS-DRG Codes by Total Annual Medicare Charges, 2015

MS-DRG Code	MS-DRG Description	Frequency	Total Charges (Millions of Dollars)	Blood Charges (Millions of Dollars)	Blood as % of Total Charges
470	Major joint replacement or reattachment of lower extremity w/o MCC	447,204	$23,792	$105	0.4%
871	Septicemia or severe sepsis w/o MV >96 hours w MCC	438,395	$21,265	$213	1.0%
853	Infectious and parasitic diseases w O.R. procedure w MCC	59,724	$8,081	$123	1.5%
291	Heart failure and shock w MCC	201,085	$7,781	$46	0.6%
460	Spinal fusion except cervical w/o MCC	75,165	$7,472	$23	0.3%
3	ECMO or trach w MV >96 hrs or PDX exc face, mouth and neck w maj O.R.	16,842	$7,467	$158	2.1%
247	PERC cardiovascular procedure with drug-eluting stent w/o MCC	85,126	$6,228	$3	0.1%
870	Septicemia or severe sepsis w MV >96 hrs	34,104	$5,383	$67	1.2%
193	Simple pneumonia and pleurisy with MCC	135,687	$5,246	$32	0.6%
329	Major small and large bowel procedures with MCC	38,789	$5,234	$76	1.5%

SOURCES: RAND analysis of the CMS AOR/BOR file from the 2016 Inpatient Prospective Payment System Final Rule. Estimates reflect CMS AOR data. Blood charges are from the "Blood Charges Within DRG" category.

common MS-DRGs with significant blood use (e.g., GI hemorrhage with complications, MS-DRG 378, with 6.6 percent of total charges associated with blood). The MS-DRGs with the largest share of total charges associated with blood include bone marrow transplant and diagnoses for leukemia and blood disorders.

Medicare updates MS-DRG payment rates annually in the Inpatient Prospective Payment System (IPPS). The payment rate for each MS-DRG is based on a base rate reflecting the costs for all Medicare discharges, a MS-DRG–specific relative weight comparing the costs for an individual MS-DRG to the Medicare average, and adjustments for changing market conditions. Hospitals are required to report charges and costs to Medicare to inform payment rate updates, including separate estimates of blood purchase and transfusion service costs.

Table 5.2
Top MS-DRG Codes by Total Blood Charges, 2015

MS-DRG Code	MS-DRG Description	Frequency	Total Charges (Millions of Dollars)	Blood Charges (Millions of Dollars)	Blood as % of Total Charges
378	GI hemorrhage w CC	141,289	$3,907	$260	6.6%
871	Septicemia or severe sepsis w/o MV >96 hrs w MCC	438,395	$21,265	$213	1.0%
3	ECMO or trach w MV >96 hrs or PDX EXC face, mouth and neck with major OR	16,842	$7,467	$158	2.1%
377	GI hemorrhage w MCC	58,688	$2,728	$157	5.7%
812	RBC disorders w/o MCC	75,238	$1,751	$151	8.6%
853	Infectious and parasitic diseases with O.R. procedure w MCC	59,724	$8,081	$123	1.5%
470	Major joint replacement or reattachment of lower extremity w/o MCC	447,204	$23,792	$105	0.4%
219	Cardiac valve and oth major cardiothoracic procedure w/o card cath w MCC	17,056	$3,502	$101	2.9%
481	Hip and femur procedures except major joint w CC	81,732	$4,297	$901	2.1%
811	RBC disorders w MCC	31,310	$1,094	$80	7.3%

SOURCES: RAND analysis of the CMS AOR/BOR file from the 2016 Inpatient Prospective Payment System Final Rule. Estimates reflect CMS AOR data. Blood costs are from the "Blood Charges Within DRG" category.

CMS updates IPPS rates using cost information that is lagged by two years. Costs are organized for reporting purposes into revenue codes, including two blood-related codes, 038x (Blood) and 039x (Blood and Component Administration, Processing and Storage). Hospitals that obtain blood at technically no charge for the product itself (only a payment for processing and related services) report using the second revenue code. This is the common reporting approach for blood supplied by ARC and other nonprofit blood centers.

It is important to note that the DRG system and IPPS cover payments to facilities, not to physicians and other providers furnishing care during the hospital stay who can separately bill Medicare under the Physician Fee Schedule (PFS). The total cost to Medicare of an inpatient stay includes the facility payment under IPPS, plus any related professional services like surgical services paid under PFS.

Table 5.3
Top MS-DRG Codes by Blood Share of Total Charges, 2015

MS-DRG Code	MS-DRG Description	Frequency	Total Charges (Millions of Dollars)	Blood Charges (Millions of Dollars)	Blood as % of Total Charges
14	Allogeneic bone marrow transplant	797	$230	$44	19.2%
834	Acute leukemia w/o major O.R. procedure w MCC	3,909	$563	$67	11.9%
836	Acute leukemia w/o major O.R. procedure w/o CC/MCC	797	$24	$3	11.1%
837	Chemo w acute leukemia as sdx or with high-dose chemo agent w MCC	1,816	$287	$32	11.1%
835	Acute leukemia w/o major O.R. procedure w CC	2,552	$155	$16	10.2%
810	Major hematol/immun diag exc sickle cell crisis and coagulation w/o CC/MCC	2,371	$58	$5	9.3%
809	Major hematol/immun diag exc sickle cell crisis and coagulation w CC	16,786	$554	$48	8.8%
812	RBC disorders w/o MCC	75,238	$1,751	$151	8.6%
808	Major hematol/immun diag exc sickle cell crisis and coagulation w MCC	7,786	$468	$38	8.1%
813	Coagulation disorders	8,192	$406	$32	7.9%

SOURCES: RAND analysis of the CMS AOR/BOR file from the 2016 Inpatient Prospective Payment System Final Rule. Estimates reflect CMS AOR data. Blood costs are from the "Blood Charges Within DRG" category.

Facility Payments for Care Delivered in the Outpatient Setting

In the HOPD setting, Medicare pays hospitals under OPPS. Individual outpatient services are identified by HCPCS codes. HCPCS codes are assigned to APCs based on clinical and resource homogeneity. The payment rate calculated for each APC applies to the related health care services grouped in the same APC. For example, Medicare makes a single payment for Level 1 Skin Procedures (APC 5051).[6] Many ancillary and supportive services—such as supplies, anesthesia, implantable devices, and some

---

[6]   CMS, "Hospital Outpatient Prospective Payment—Final Rule with Comment Period and Final CY2016 Payment Rates," Baltimore, Md., 2016b.

drugs[7]—are bundled into the APC payment. However, blood products, transfusion services, and some other services, such as some drugs and preventive services, are paid separately and are assigned their own APCs. APC payment rates (including payment rates for blood APCs) are updated annually to account for inflation and changes in labor input prices. There are special adjustments on individual payments to rural hospitals and to some cancer hospitals.

As a result, in the outpatient hospital setting, hospitals are paid more directly for blood acquisition by Medicare rather than based on bundled average costs, as in the inpatient setting. Hospitals do not face the same financial incentives with respect to blood in the ambulatory setting as they do in the inpatient setting. Overall, however, only 10 percent to 20 percent of blood transfusions occur in the outpatient setting. There have been changes to Medicare's treatment of blood and transfusion services in the hospital outpatient setting. For example, in the 2016 OPPS, CMS bundled a set of transfusion laboratory APCs—but not blood product APCs—that were previously separately paid into the rates for other APCs. In 2016, CMS also expanded the number of comprehensive APCs, which package payment for adjunctive items, services, and procedures (including blood and blood products) into the most costly primary procedure under OPPS at the claim level.

Payments for Professional Services

Medicare pays physicians and other health professionals using a separate PFS. In most cases, routine transfusion services are included in the facility payment (either through IPPS or OPPS), and no additional professional payment is necessary. However, in cases where physicians are involved in interpreting test results or are present during the transfusion service, they are able to bill for separate payment.

Other Public Financing

Both Medicare and Medicaid operate Disproportionate Share Hospital (DSH) programs in which the federal government and states (in the case of Medicaid DSH) make separate payments to hospitals serving a disproportionate share of Medicaid enrollees and the uninsured. Medicaid DSH payments alone were $15 billion in FY 2015.[8] The ACA put in place significant reductions in DSH payments to reflect the shrinking uninsured population. For Medicaid, these reductions were delayed until FY 2017. Other state and local government funding help offset hospital-operating expenses. In the outpatient setting, HRSA awards grants to federally quali-

---

7   Relatively inexpensive drugs (i.e., below a $90 per diem threshold in the 2016 OPPS) are bundled into APC payments.

8   HHS, "Medicaid Program; Final FY 2013 and Preliminary FY 2015 Disproportionate Share Hospital Allotments, and Final FY 2013 and Preliminary FY 2015 Institutions for Mental Diseases Disproportionate Share Hospital Limits," Federal Register, Vol. 81, No. 21, February 2016.

fied health centers (FQHCs) and other providers to expand health care services for underserved populations. HRSA's FY 2017 budget request included $5.1 billion for primary health care focusing on grants to FQHCs and additional resources for HIV/AIDS grantees and maternal and child health grantees.[9]

Cost-Sharing

Patient cost-sharing represents a fraction of the revenue received by hospitals from payers. Patients covered by Medicare Part A (hospital insurance) pay an annual deductible and cost-sharing for inpatient stays beyond a certain number of threshold days. Patients covered by Medicare Part B (medical insurance) pay a premium, a modest deductible, and 20 percent of the Medicare allowed amount for services. Medicare has a separate blood deductible that applies to blood used in the inpatient setting (Part A) and outpatient setting (Part B) where patients are responsible for paying for the first three units of blood used in their care. However, CMS interprets the blood deductible to apply only when the provider purchases blood for the patient—and not when the provider receives blood from a blood center charging only for processing and other services, which is far more common than direct purchase.

Payment in the Broader Health Care System

In large part, other U.S. public insurers (such as state Medicaid programs, the DoD TRICARE program, and VHA) and private insurers follow Medicare's approach to payment for inpatient and outpatient care. Payment rates for specific inpatient stays or outpatient services, however, do vary across payers, with Medicaid rates in general falling below Medicare and other public payer rates, and commercial rates in general above public rates.

Strengths of Status Quo Payment Arrangements

Our conversations with stakeholders and our other research highlighted important strengths of the current prevailing payment arrangements. Most importantly, current payment policy incentivizes hospitals to be cost-conscious users and purchasers of blood (and other inputs into care), thus lowering health care spending. Declining prices and reports of robust competition suggest that Medicare's payment policies are achieving their cost containment goals, at least with respect to blood. Providing hospitals with an incentive to pursue lower blood prices aggressively may be one important catalyst for changes in market structure among blood centers, particularly consolidation among smaller blood centers to enable them to compete on price with larger-scale entities like ARC.

---

[9]   HRSA, "FY 2017 Budget Overview," Rockville, Md., last reviewed March 2016.

Impacts of Payment Policy on Blood Centers

Through our interviews with blood centers and other stakeholder groups, we identi-fied three ways that payment policy could place stress on blood centers. First, interview participants highlighted a potential disconnect between payments for inpatient care and the actual use of blood. Hospitals receive the same payment under DRG-based payment arrangements regardless of whether blood is used (and regardless of how other inputs into care, such as hospital equipment, clinical labor, and medical devices, are used). Therefore, hospitals have a financial incentive to limit the utilization of blood, and as a result, current payment arrangements help control the contribution of blood to total health care spending. But paying hospitals a single amount per discharge makes it challenging to develop and implement payment policies that target a single input into care, such as blood. For example, it would be challenging under a DRG-based payment to persuade hospitals on financial grounds alone to pay higher prices for pathogen-reduced blood because this increases hospital costs without a matching change in rev-enue (at least in the short term until IPPS rates are updated). Even if payers increased rates to accommodate new products or higher blood costs, there is no guarantee that hospitals—the recipients of the additional payments—would pass on the payments to blood centers.

Second, interview participants noted that lagged updates in payment rates for health care services can, in some cases, place short-term financial stress on blood cen-ters bearing the costs of new required testing or other factors leading to higher produc-tion costs, particularly when blood centers are unwilling to renegotiate contracts with hospitals. For example, the IPPS relative weights used to update payment for specific MS-DRGs are updated using cost data lagged by two years. In other words, if hospi-tals' costs for blood-intensive MS-DRGs were to increase at a higher rate than costs for other MS-DRGs (e.g., by 10 percent this year compared with lower growth for other MS-DRGs), the rates paid to hospitals would not reflect the new payment relativities for two more years. It is not clear whether blood centers or hospitals are more impacted by this lag. If blood centers are not able or willing to pass on the additional produc-tion costs to hospitals—for example, if they do not want to risk their hospital buyers considering alternative blood suppliers—then blood centers will not report additional costs to payers, and existing payment rates will persist. In this scenario, blood centers must cope with smaller margins or losses per unit on an ongoing basis. However, if blood centers do pass on the additional product costs to hospitals, then hospitals will have higher acquisition costs for the two years until payment rates are updated. It is likely that there is heterogeneity across markets, blood centers, and hospitals in terms of how such a scenario would play out. Some of our interview participants indicated that, while they have clauses in their contracts with hospitals to raise or renegotiate prices with hospitals in the event of new FDA-required testing or other major market changes, they had never exercised this option for fear of upsetting their buyers. Other interview participants reported increasing prices charged to hospitals to cover, for example, new tests.

Finally, some interview participants noted that when payments are made directly for blood (e.g., under OPPS), payment amounts are not always specific to highly differentiated blood products. This could lead to an undersupply of specific products where production costs are higher than the payment rate and an oversupply of products where production costs are relatively low compared with the payment rate. In the 2016 OPPS final rule, new APCs for pathogen-reduced plasma and platelets were established, and CMS noted the intention "in future rulemaking to evaluate the set of HCPCS P-codes and propose revisions that may be necessary to create a current and robust code set for blood products."[10]

Payment Policy Alternatives

Each of these issues has the potential to place stress on blood centers. This section discusses a set of alternative payment policies that could mitigate these pressures in the short term, if this is the policy goal. It is important to consider the status quo as an important policy option, given the advantages in terms of incentives for price competition noted earlier.

We introduce a framework to describe a range of changes to payment policies related to blood; describe a set of payment policy alternatives identified through our primary data collection effort, literature review, and review of payment policy in other health care sectors; and then estimate the effects of three alternative payment models.

Framework

We developed a framework (Table 5.4) to categorize policies along two dimensions. The first dimension indicates the target of the payment and policy: either hospitals—mirroring current arrangements in which payments flow to hospitals—or blood centers directly. While direct payments from payers to blood centers are currently rare, there are important analogues elsewhere in the U.S. health care system, such as direct payments to specialty pharmacies for drugs that are ultimately used in physician offices and payments to freestanding organ procurement organizations for organs that are ultimately transplanted in a hospital, that suggest such an arrangement might be possible even for Medicare (where statutory language restricts payment to specific provider categories). Private payers might have more flexibility in paying blood centers directly. The second dimension of the framework arranges potential policies in three categories: pass-through policies, where payment for blood is separated from currently bundled payments like DRG-based payments for inpatient care; subsidies, where payers

---

[10] CMS, undated-b.

Table 5.4
Framework for Considering Payment Policies

Target	Tool		
	DRG Pass-Through	Supplement	Subsidy
Hospital	Separate blood payments to hospitals	Per-unit supplement paid to hospitals	Subsidy paid to hospitals
Blood center	Separate blood payments to blood centers	Per-unit supplement paid to blood centers	Subsidy paid to blood centers

make lump-sum transfers to blood centers or hospitals; and supplements, where payers increase per-unit payment rates.

This framework covers payment arrangements for health care services in the traditional sense—for example, pass-through payments or supplemental payments to hospitals. However, it expands into the broader areas of financing and investments in public health not specifically related to payment for health care services (e.g., subsidies paid to blood centers). We view this broad framework as appropriate, given the range of policy alternatives that could improve the sustainability of the blood system.

Policy Alternatives

The following sections discuss a set of six alternative payment policies, including important design issues and likely impacts of each. These six policies map to the six cells in Table 5.4, as indicated in parentheses in the following list:

1. DRG pass-through for blood (DRG pass-through paid to hospitals)
2. Direct payment to blood centers (DRG pass-through paid to blood centers)
3. Blood technology supplemental payment (per-unit supplement paid to hospitals)
4. Blood technology adoption subsidies (per-unit supplement paid to blood centers)
5. Disproportionate blood share model (subsidy paid to hospitals)
6. Grants to blood centers (subsidy paid to blood centers).

Some of the policy alternatives—including the DRG pass-through and the disproportionate share hospital-like policy for blood—have been discussed in public forums[11] and were raised by stakeholders during interviews. We developed other policy alternatives—including the blood technology adoption subsidy policy—after synthesizing feedback from interviews and other study activities.

---

[11] HHS, Office of the HIV/AIDS and Infectious Disease Policy, "Recommendations of the 47th Meeting of the ACBTSA, November 9–10, 2015," November 2015.

The bold headings under each of the six policies in the following sections are our summary of potential advantages and disadvantages of policies informed by our expert opinion, review of the literature, and conversations with stakeholders. In most cases we did not identify specific studies or analyses supporting these arguments directly. The likely effects of each policy alternative hinge on a set of detailed decisions that would need to be made by HHS on how the policy is designed and implemented—for example, specific payment amounts, eligibility criteria, or rate-updating provisions—and we do not describe alternatives at this level of detail.

Furthermore, it is important to note that several of these policy alternatives result in differential treatment or additional funding for blood or specific stakeholders in the blood system relative to policy and payment for suppliers of other critical inputs into the health care system. CMS and HHS might be concerned about a "slippery slope" when considering the feasibility of justifying and implementing these policy alternatives. While we note specific challenges in design and implementation in the following sections, we do not comment extensively on political or other pressures that might determine whether these policy alternatives are feasible.

1. DRG Pass-Through for Blood

Because episode-based payments such as those in the DRG system are fixed regardless of the number or type of blood units transfused, hospitals are not fully compensated for atypical care that they provide to patients requiring above-average volume or intensity of care and inputs into care, including blood relative to other patients assigned to the same MS-DRG. Separating blood payments from per-stay DRG payments could—depending on how the pass-through is designed—remove some of the financial incentives for hospitals to actively control transfusion rates and facilitate quicker updates to payment in response to changes in cost. In addition, separate accounting for blood could increase the salience of blood to hospital administrators and policymakers.

Currently, CMS uses pass-through payments for some medical devices and expensive drugs in OPPS and for blood factors in the inpatient and outpatient settings. In both cases, the pass-through is budget neutral—in other words, the additional Medicare spending on pass-through drugs and devices results in lower payments per MS-DRG—with payments via the pass-through based on hospital acquisition costs. The blood-specific pass-through policy alternative described in this section removes blood purchase costs—including payments to nonprofit blood centers for processing and services—from DRG payments. Medicare would then separately pay hospitals for blood at a cost-based (i.e., based on reported or empirically derived costs) or rate-based (i.e., based on a rate set considering costs and possibly other factors) per-unit amount and continue paying for inpatient stays under the DRG system, minus the reduction from the pass-through. The distinction between a cost-based or rate-based payment is important and will determine whether hospitals will retain any incentive to control blood use.

Separating blood payments may increase hospital coding accuracy. Currently, there is concern that hospitals do not document all blood inputs used in furnishing care in their systems to transmit cost information to CMS for IPPS rate updates. Separating blood payments via a pass-through could improve reporting by hospitals because they would only be paid for units recorded in claims data paid under fee-for-service.

A blood pass-through could reduce efficiency and incentives for cost containment. Under DRGs, providers are reimbursed at a fixed rate per discharge based on diagnosis, treatment, and type of discharge. As a result, the DRG system provides a financial incentive for hospitals to reduce unnecessary treatments and procedures. Removing blood from DRG payments could reduce incentives for hospital cost control for blood. To the extent that blood costs drive hospital efforts to reduce use—for example, through patient blood management programs—a blood pass-through could increase transfusion volume.

A blood pass-through could increase or decrease payments to blood centers. Under the current model, hospitals contract with blood centers to acquire blood—there is no direct reimbursement from CMS to blood centers. If a pass-through is intended to benefit blood centers, the resulting separate payments for blood to hospitals must somehow spill over to blood centers. While separate payment might increase the salience of blood to hospital administrators, it is not clear whether this increased attention would increase or decrease the payments to blood centers resulting from negotiations between hospitals and centers. For example, under a blood pass-through with cost-based payment, hospitals that had negotiated prices above the national average might be prompted by the pass-through to look for lower-cost suppliers. The most likely general effect is that a blood pass-through would increase utilization by hospitals, resulting in higher revenue for blood centers under the typical consignment model without changes in per-unit price.

Payments based on average cost will not cover all costs. CMS would need to set a per-unit price for blood under this policy. One alternative is to use cost-based prices from the OPPS outpatient hospital fee schedule. This type of average cost-based payment would give larger margins to hospitals able to purchase blood at relatively low rates, while hospitals buying blood at relatively higher rates would lose money on blood. One alternative model—cost-based reimbursement (i.e., passing through hospital-specific costs rather than an average rate)—is rarely used in the U.S. health care system because of the lack of cost-control incentives. However, this model has the advantage of ensuring that hospitals would not lose money per unit of blood transfused.

Pass-through rates can be updated differently or more often. CMS could update cost-based blood payment rates under the pass-through more frequently and with more-current data. As a result, hospitals could receive higher payment rates more quickly in response to changes in blood costs.

The net effects of such a policy would be small. We expect little change in hospital or blood center revenue in aggregate if payment rates under a blood pass-through would mirror the current market rates for blood (i.e., the costs paid by hospitals to acquire blood). A cost-based pass-through would, however, increase blood-related revenue for hospitals with high transfusion rates and decrease blood-related revenue for hospitals with low transfusion rates. In other words, a pass-through better targets payments for blood toward hospitals with the largest blood costs. CMS could set other—perhaps higher—rates for blood. In this case, aggregate revenue to hospitals with high transfusion rates would also increase. It is not clear whether these revenues would be passed on to blood centers.

2. Direct Payment to Blood Centers

This variant of the first policy alternative involves carving payment for blood out of the DRG system and paying blood centers directly. Services related to blood—for example, storage and transfusion services—could still be bundled into DRG payments to hospitals. In the Medicare context, the feasibility of this policy hinges on whether CMS could consider blood centers as health care providers.

Medicare's payment approach for organ transplants offers a helpful analogy for this policy alternative. Medicare pays for transplants through IPPS as with other inpatient stays. Transplanting hospitals obtain organs through organ procurement entities affiliated with the hospital or from independent organ procurement organizations (IOPOs). Medicare requires IOPOs to report their costs and revenue associated with organ procurement for Medicare patients and reconciles payment with IOPOs annually. In other words, if an IOPO reports higher costs related to procuring organs transplanted in Medicare beneficiaries than the IOPO received in revenue from hospitals, then the IOPO receives an additional payment from Medicare.

Setting payment rates is challenging and could disproportionately benefit some blood centers. Because this policy involves paying blood centers rather than hospitals, it would be inappropriate to use OPPS or other existing payment systems. CMS could choose to pay a fixed rate to blood centers based on production costs (possibly with regional adjustments). This would result in a single per-unit payment rate for different blood products that would result in higher margins for blood centers with relatively low marginal costs and smaller margins for blood centers with higher marginal costs. As an alternative, CMS could pay a blood-center–specific rate based on cost or reconcile costs against revenues, as CMS does for IOPOs. Because of economies of scale, blood centers could have dramatically different production costs based on the volume of blood collected and processed. Furthermore, some centers have more aggressive technology adoption policies than others, increasing short-term costs. In either case, CMS would need to develop an approach to establishing initial payment rates and updating payment rates over time.

This policy ensures that increases in CMS reimbursement for blood and blood products would go directly to blood centers, rather than hospitals. Assuming that CMS payment rates keep pace with changes in production costs, payments directly to blood centers would ensure that blood centers would not be penalized for increases in production costs—for example, costs associated with new required tests.

Taking financial risk out of hospitals' hands may increase blood utilization. CMS utilizes bundled payments to control costs by providing financial incentives. When blood centers are paid directly by CMS, hospitals have fewer incentives to manage blood utilization, and, therefore, the number of units transfused can increase.

Blood centers may face a new administrative burden. Blood centers would need to begin billing Medicare for blood units used in the course of care or accounting for aggregate costs and revenues related to blood used by Medicare patients. This is a major, and possibly insurmountable, health IT and coordination challenge, given that blood is used by separate organizations, hospitals, and blood centers, some of which have no way of knowing how blood is used in clinical care.

The net effects of such a policy hinge on design details. The specific effects of this policy hinge in large part on the details of the payment arrangements put in place between payers and blood centers. As with the blood pass-through under the existing DRG system, we expect little change in hospital or blood center revenue under this policy if payments are based on production costs. Under a purely rate-based approach, however, blood centers with high production costs could receive less revenue under this policy than they had negotiated with hospitals previously. This could, in turn, spur cost-cutting or exit of blood centers with high production costs.

3. Blood Technology Supplemental Payment

In 2000, Congress took steps to ensure that Medicare beneficiaries would have timely access to new, breakthrough technologies that, absent any additional payments, would be inadequately paid for under the existing DRG amount. The intent of the additional payments was to bridge the recalibration delay (e.g., updating rates using cost data with a two-year lag) by providing a temporary payment mechanism for the use of new technologies in addition to the DRG payment amount the hospital would otherwise receive. The new technology add-on payments (NTAPs) were to be provided until CMS had inpatient claims data for DRG rate-setting that reflected the added costs of the new technology.

Today, for a technology to be eligible for an NTAP, it must meet the following three conditions: The technology must be new, which CMS generally defines as within two to three years following FDA approval or market introduction, if later; the existing DRG payment for the service involving the technology must be inadequate, as demonstrated by meeting thresholds calculated annually by CMS; and the technology must be a substantial clinical improvement over existing services.

The NTAP formula established by CMS requires Medicare and hospitals to share in the financial risk of providing costly new technologies. The NTAP amount paid for an individual discharge is equal to the lesser of 50 percent of the amount by which the total covered costs of the case exceed the DRG payment or 50 percent of the costs of the new technology.

In the context of blood, NTAP could be applied to help pay for new required or underused tests or such products as pathogen-reduced blood. Or, as a close alternative, a new program similar to NTAP could focus specifically on blood-related technologies. In either case, this policy alternative could apply to new FDA-mandated technologies.

Supplemental payments can incentivize early adoption of new technologies and safety measures. Supplemental payments that are available shortly after a technology is introduced could significantly increase adoption rates. This could be especially important for tests not yet mandated by FDA or new product lines, such as pathogen-reduced blood, not yet widely used in the health care system.

Integrating value into the policy design is challenging. The NTAP program uses value as one criterion to determine whether a technology is eligible for a supplemental payment. While a blood-specific policy could do the same, it is more challenging to evaluate value in the context of blood than in many other inputs into health care for a range of reasons, including the public health importance of blood and the lack of substitutes.

Current CMS criteria for new technologies may not be applicable to blood. Through regulatory provisions, CMS has structured the NTAP program criteria to ensure that only a subset of new technologies qualifies. Most notably, technologies must be found to offer substantial clinical improvement over existing technologies to qualify. This requirement may be one reason that relatively few NTAP applications have been approved (19 of 53 applications from 2001 to 2015), compared with initial projections by Congress and CMS.[12]

Supplemental payments targeting new technology would increase health care spending and could benefit blood centers. Based on our interviews with blood center leadership and other stakeholders, we estimate that the incremental production cost of a Zika virus screening or a similar test is $20 per unit. With 14.4 million RBC units in available supply in 2013[13] and an assumption that 80 percent of blood is used in the inpatient setting and 60 percent of inpatient care is provided to Medicare beneficiaries, a supplemental payment policy in which Medicare bears all of the new technology cost would add $138.2 million in Medicare payments to hospitals.[14] It is not clear what proportion of this additional spending, if any, would be passed on to blood centers.

---

[12] J. Hernandez, S. Machacz, and J. Robinson, "U.S. Hospital Payment Adjustments for Innovative Technology Lag Behind Those in Germany, France, and Japan," *Health Affairs*, Vol. 34, No. 2, 2015.

[13] Chung et al., 2016.

[14] While NTAP was budget neutral when it was introduced, the 2003 Medicare Modernization Act removed this requirement. See A. Clyde, L. Bockstedt, J. Farkas, and C. Jackson, "Experience with Medicare's New Technology Add-On Payment Program," *Health Affairs*, Vol. 27, No. 6, 2008.

4. Blood Technology Adoption Subsidies

Building on the prior policy, subsidy payments (either framed as an outright subsidy or a per-unit payment) could flow from payers or the government to blood centers directly as an incentive for the adoption of new technology, such as pathogen testing.

Subsidies to blood centers may be more feasible from the government rather than from public payers, such as Medicare. As noted earlier, Medicare is constrained in terms of the entities that it considers as providers for the purposes of payment. One advantage of a broader technology adoption subsidy is that payments could flow from the government more broadly—for example, through the procurement authority of BARDA, where there is a clear public health or preparedness case in favor of technology adoption.

Subsidies to blood centers directly target the entities bearing new production costs. Unlike payments targeted to hospitals, subsidy payments to blood centers directly reimburse the entities that integrate many new technologies and testing requirements into their production processes.

Identifying qualifying technologies is challenging. One option is to include tests or other process innovations required by FDA in the subsidy scheme. Other technologies—for example, pathogen-reduced blood—might qualify under the recommendation of the HHS secretary.

Technology-based subsidies to blood centers would increase government spending and would benefit blood centers. As in the prior policy, subsidies would increase payer or government payments for blood. In contrast with the prior policy, however, subsidies paid directly to blood centers would improve the financial situation for blood suppliers.

5. Disproportionate Blood Share Model

Both Medicaid and Medicare DSH programs result in subsidies paid to individual hospitals. For Medicaid DSH, the payment amounts to individual hospitals are left up to the state. Medicare DSH follows a formulaic approach to allocating payment amounts. A Disproportionate Blood Share Hospital (DBSH) policy for blood would target subsidies to hospitals with disproportionate costs associated with purchasing and using blood, such as trauma centers and hospitals offering hematology and oncology services. These payments would help offset the difference between the proportion of payment for blood under current payment arrangements and the actual blood-related costs borne by these hospitals.

DBSH would provide financial support to institutions bearing the highest blood purchase costs. It is not clear whether these additional resources would be used to furnish additional services in the specific service lines that qualify a hospital for DBSH (e.g., trauma care or hematology and oncology), used to cross-subsidize other service lines, or passed through to blood centers.

Developing eligibility and allotment criteria would be challenging. One approach is to target outlier hospitals with blood costs well above the contribution of blood to current MS-DRG rates.

It is not clear who would finance a DBSH program. Medicare and Medicaid are two potential sources for financing, although private insurers would also benefit from such a program and could contribute.

Setting subsidy amounts is arbitrary. The payers or other government entities financing the DBSH program would need to determine subsidy amounts. Given the challenges in cost accounting for inpatient care in particular, this process will be somewhat imprecise. One option is to transfer, at most, the difference between recorded blood costs at each hospital and the average blood costs for DRGs (where blood charges are common).

DBSH could erode incentives for blood cost control. Separately financing excess blood spending could erode incentives for hospitals to keep blood acquisition costs and blood-related service costs low.

A DBSH policy would likely lead to a modest increase in blood use and health care spending. Although the effects of a disproportionate share program for blood hinge on design details, it is likely that such a program would encourage some hospitals that were already significant users of blood to increase utilization. Other hospitals—for example, those contemplating moves into blood-intensive service lines—could also increase use as a result of this policy. The contributors to DBSH program financing would make additional transfers to hospitals beyond current payments, thereby increasing health care spending.

6. Grants to Blood Centers

Although not specifically a payment policy, this last alternative accomplishes directly what multiple stakeholders said they hoped to accomplish through changes in payment: increasing revenue to blood centers. If this is the policy goal, direct subsidies to blood centers in the form of grants to support operations may be easier to implement than many payment alternatives. A grant program could mirror HRSA's significant financing of the primary care safety net, including FQHCs. There are also important analogies to government investments in surge capacity and preparedness.

Blood center grants would not interfere with payment arrangements for health care services. The current payment arrangements for blood and health care services involving blood could continue uninterrupted.

The government would need to develop eligibility requirements. The government could decide whether to consider production costs, revenue received from hospitals, or other factors when designing eligibility criteria. Financial information submitted to HHS by applicants may improve the government's understanding of challenges facing blood centers. As an alternative, all blood centers could be eligible to receive grants in proportion to their costs or volume.

Grants may undermine market forces. Depending on the eligibility criteria that are ultimately developed and on how the grant program is administered, grants to blood centers may dull incentives for efficiency in terms of production and distribution.

Conclusions

The complex payment arrangements for health care services in the United States typically do not treat blood as a separately paid product or service. Furthermore, payments are made to hospitals rather than to blood centers (as is the case for various inputs into care, including medical devices, some drugs, labor, and other supplies). As a result, mitigating financial stresses on blood centers, if this is a policy goal, through changes in payment arrangements is challenging.

Some policy alternatives—for example, supplemental payments tied to technologies or general subsidies paid by the government directly to blood centers—would not necessarily disrupt any of the current payment arrangements in place between payers and hospitals. Other policy alternatives mentioned by stakeholders—for example, a blood pass-through in IPPS—would pay hospitals in a more-targeted way based on their blood utilization while allowing more-frequent updates to payment rates and increasing the salience of blood as an input into health care. The likely impacts of a pass-through hinge on a set of important design decisions, such as whether payment is based on costs or another rate.

It is worth reemphasizing the success of current payment arrangements in promoting price competition between blood centers and cost control in aggregate among hospitals. Many of the policies outlined earlier would distort market incentives for blood centers. In the long term, current policy might serve as a catalyst for consolidation between blood centers as economies of scale become important to offer lower unit prices. Depending on whether and how consolidation occurs, policymakers might be concerned in the future about supplier power and rising blood costs.

CHAPTER SIX

The Value of an Available Blood Supply

Blood—like pharmaceuticals, medical devices, and practitioner labor—is an important input in lifesaving surgical procedures and treatments. Hospitals and patients benefit from having blood available for routine procedures but also derive value in having blood readily available in the event of an emergency. Some have referred to the latter value as an insurance value of blood, as it reflects a certain risk or uncertainty in the demand for blood. In other words, individuals cannot predict when they might need blood, and hospitals, although perhaps better at forecasting blood needs overall, may also unexpectedly need more blood than they have on hand.

In this chapter, we describe the value of available blood even when the blood is not being immediately used. In other words, society, hospitals, and patients face uncertainty about when and how much blood they require, but these stakeholders derive value from having blood available. We draw heavily on economic theory to describe potential market mechanisms to address the uncertainty.

There is risk or uncertainty that individual hospitals might not have enough blood in the event of an emergency or that they might have to ration blood (e.g., by canceling or rescheduling elective surgeries or treatments when blood was not available). More broadly, there is also society-level risk that events could occur that would threaten the blood supply's ability to meet demand in an emergency. At both levels, there is uncertainty that precludes hospitals and society at large from knowing the full range of possible disruptions to the blood supply that could cause a shortage. Even when possible disruptions are identified, the probability and timing of such events occurring is also uncertain.

In this chapter, we describe how the market has historically addressed and currently addresses uncertainty, and we discuss possible alternative market mechanisms that could mitigate risks. To achieve these aims, we briefly describe supply chain costs and transactions in the blood system, which do not necessarily reflect the value of blood, and discuss how blood might be considered a public good.

Price of Blood

We first note that it is important to distinguish between the price paid for a unit of blood and the value that a patient, hospital, or society receives from the same unit. The equilibrium or market clearing price does not necessarily reflect the full value that a patient, hospital, or society receives from buying that unit of blood. In fact, people might be willing to pay considerably more than the actual price paid; in economics, this positive difference between what the buyer would have been willing to pay (also known as the reservation price) and what the buyer actually pays is referred to as a consumer surplus. Thus, trying to assign a value to a unit of blood using transaction data (such as purchase prices) is not straightforward. Using the market price as an estimate will be misleading, as patients and hospitals likely value blood more than the price paid indicates. At the same time, other approaches to estimating value (such as those used in cost-effectiveness research) rely on willingness-to-pay measures that are difficult to translate for a unit of lifesaving blood.

The price of blood reflects conditions in both the supply and demand sides of the market (i.e., the production and distribution of blood by blood centers and the purchase and use of blood by hospitals). Although the market price does reveal information about costs of production, it is likely less than the benefit that patients derive from receiving a unit of blood. As such, the market price suggests at least a lower bound of the benefit of blood, in dollar terms, to patients and society. The following sections describe both sides of the market for blood and prevailing prices.

Supply of Blood

The supply chain for blood products has several stages, as described in Chapter One. Here, we briefly highlight key cost drivers along the supply chain. Collection costs to recruit, screen, and draw blood include a wide range of staff, capital (facilities and equipment), and logistical supports. Other variable costs include medical supplies necessary for collection and processing, disposal of biohazardous waste, efforts to handle adverse reactions, and post-donation donor follow-up, as needed.[1]

Testing, whether outsourced or performed in house, is also a significant component of costs for blood centers. Often, this includes transportation and other logistical support service costs in addition to laboratory costs. Testing for blood type includes testing for standard ABO blood groupings and Rhesus factors, which also requires reagents and specialized equipment.[2] Costs for matching blood include extended compatibility testing (antigen typing) and human lymphocyte antigen matching, although

---

[1] Cost of Blood Consensus Conference, 2005.

[2] Cost of Blood Consensus Conference, 2005; Arianna Simonetti, Richard A. Forshee, Steven A. Anderson, and Mark Walderhaug, "A Stock and Flow Simulation Model of the U.S. Blood Supply," *Transfusion*, Vol. 54, No. 3, Part 2, 2014, pp. 828–838.

this type of cost tends to be incurred only for certain patients.[3] Some testing and cross-matching can be done using computers, thus avoiding the costly laboratory testing.

There are also costs associated with specific processing procedures, such as freezing or glycerolizing red cells, leukoreduction, and separating out special components (e.g., plasma cryoprecipitate).[4] Finally, there are various logistical and transportation costs, including costs to manage inventories.[5]

Previous research has shown that the majority of the direct costs of blood are typically in collection at around $150 to $250 per unit in the United States (or about 20 percent to 30 percent of total costs).[6] Pre-transfusion processes and patient blood testing are 5 percent to 12 percent and 8 percent to 12 percent of total costs in the United States, respectively. These figures are somewhat dated and not representative, but blood center cost data are not typically publicly available, making it difficult to estimate the margins for blood centers precisely.

Hospital Purchase Prices and Quantity Supplied

Hospitals negotiate payment rates with blood centers for individual products. These negotiations also determine a range of logistics and service provisions. Based on the most recent findings from the NBCUS survey, the average price that hospitals paid blood centers for a single leuko-reduced RBC unit in 2013 was $226 (see Figure 5.2). However, there was significant variation in price, which ranged from $166 to $440. Although prices have trended downward over time, most significantly in the past decade, it is difficult to ascertain from these summary statistics the extent to which hospitals or blood centers are bearing the cost of uncertainty in the market.

Hospitals also face a variety of costs related to blood; while there is a great deal of focus on blood purchase costs (i.e., the purchase of blood components from suppliers), there are additional costs for hospitals related to preparing blood for transfusion. Transfusions involve costs for on-site storage, pre-transfusion preparation, transfusion administration and follow-up, and long-term tracking. These include costs for labor, as well as equipment, supplies, IT infrastructure, and physical space.[7] Blood acquisition costs account for less than 1 percent of all hospital costs in the United States; however,

---

[3]   Cost of Blood Consensus Conference, 2005.

[4]   Cost of Blood Consensus Conference, 2005.

[5]   Cost of Blood Consensus Conference, 2005.

[6]   Aryeh Shander, Axel Hofmann, Sherri Ozawa, Oliver M Theusinger, Hans Gombotz, and Donat R Spahn. "Activity-Based Costs of Blood Transfusions in Surgical Patients at Four Hospitals," *Transfusion*, Vol. 50, No. 4, 2010, pp. 753–765.

[7]   R. W. Toner, L. Pizzi, B. Leas, S. K. Ballas, A. Quigley, and N. I. Goldfarb, "Costs to Hospitals of Acquiring and Processing Blood in the U.S.: A Survey of Hospital-Based Blood Banks and Transfusion Services," *Applied Health Economics and Health Policy*, Vol. 9, No. 1, 2011, pp. 29–37; D. R. Spahn and L. T. Goodnough, "Alternatives to Blood Transfusion," *Lancet*, Vol. 381, No. 9880, May 25, 2013, pp. 1855–1865.

charges for blood and transfusion-related activities represent approximately 4 percent of total hospital costs.[8]

Hospital and Blood Center Transactions

Next, we describe the typical contractual arrangements between hospitals and blood centers and discuss historical evidence from events that lead to an unexpected decrease in the number of donors or increase in the number of patients needing blood.

Hospitals typically contract with blood centers that agree to provide a certain quantity of routine units of blood at a given price. Hospitals tend to pay for blood, however, only when it is used (a consignment-type model). Some have argued that hospitals and society are receiving an insurance value in having excess blood on hand in case they need it, without actually having to pay for that value.

Empirically proving whether this is true is not straightforward. To examine whether it is true, we must first distinguish between hospitals having enough routine units on hand and having enough emergency or "stat" units in case of an unexpected event. Hospitals tend to be fairly accurate at predicting the quantity of units needed for routine use. Moreover, the ability to shift around elective surgeries, for example, allows hospitals to absorb some variation in blood needed for both routine *and* emergency use. This might be one reason that there is little empirical evidence that surgeries are canceled or rescheduled because of lack of blood. One hospital informant suggested that, in fact, few elective surgeries require blood, so although some surgeries requiring blood might be rescheduled, this may not occur very often in practice. In addition, hospitals still have incentives to avoid delays caused by a lack of blood; rescheduling surgeries requires additional labor, displaces other hospital care, and potentially imposes costs on the patients being rescheduled. In a 2003 study that collected daily supply levels of 26 transfusion services sites that purchased blood from suppliers and three blood centers, researchers found no evidence of systematic postponement or cancelation of elective and nonelective surgeries caused by the lack of blood products.[9]

The second concern of having enough units available for an emergency— although more difficult for hospitals to predict—has not historically been a significant problem for the blood system as a whole. In September 2015, FDA issued a requirement for blood manufacturers with more than a 10-percent market share to notify FDA about potential disruptions to their supply of blood and blood components.[10] Other voluntary efforts to monitor blood supply at the regional level have been taken by ABC (through its BASIS system) and AABB, which manages the Interorganiza-

---

[8]   Macpherson et al., 2007.

[9]   Nightingale et al., 2003.

[10]   Nightingale et al., 2003.

tional Task Force on Domestic Disasters and Acts of Terrorism. These initiatives enable information-sharing, blood supply monitoring, and temporary resolutions for short-falls of particular blood components. Removing excess capacity from the market, however, may prevent such responsiveness in the future.

Public health emergencies, including mass casualty events, can affect the blood supply by reducing the number of eligible donors (shock to blood supply), increasing the number of patients needing blood immediately (shock to blood demand), or imposing logistical challenges that may hamper the movement of blood through the system. Although we do not have data to investigate how these shocks affect the market price of blood or the extent to which that price captures the value of blood, examining how the blood system responds to these shocks can shed light on the extent to which there is market failure (i.e., where the quantity demanded does not meet the quantity supplied).

If we view the demand for blood as relatively inelastic—that is, not sensitive to changes in the price—then any event that reduces the supply of blood should be accompanied by an increase in price. Without an increase in market price, we would expect to observe shortages or a reduction in supplier margins if they were tapping their excess capacity to meet the rise in demand. Similarly, any event that increases the demand for blood would also result in a higher short-term equilibrium market price. Thus, we can examine historical shocks to both the supply and demand sides to assess how frequently blood shortages occurred. If shocks did not occur or very rarely occurred, then we might conclude that one or several of three things are happening: (1) Centers, hospitals, and the U.S. government are already investing enough resources into spare capacity to cover shocks (i.e., purchasing enough "insurance"); (2) shocks might have been mild or infrequent; or (3) blood centers may have maintained large amounts of spare capacity because of their slow reaction to falling demand. As centers reduce this spare capacity or as demand increases, the system's lack of a mechanism to pay for "insurance" may become suddenly apparent as previously manageable shocks become unmanageable. Next, we discuss previous empirical evidence on these potential sources of a shortage that would threaten the U.S. blood supply.

Supply-Side Shocks

The median daily stock of blood has been estimated at approximately six to seven days (Nightingale, 2003)[11] and has been on the lower end of this range more recently. Studies using simulation models to estimate the effects of shocks or disruptions to the blood supply from reduced donations have shown a very resilient blood system that can handle shorter-term disruptions, such as influenza pandemics.[12] One study suggests

---

[11] Nightingale et al., 2003.

[12] Ming-Wen An, Nicholas G. Reich, Stephen O. Crawford, Ron Brookmeyer, Thomas A. Louis, and Kenrad E. Nelson, "A Stochastic Simulator of a Blood Product Donation Environment with Demand Spikes and Supply

that increased recruitment efforts, depending on timing, can offset reduced supply from pandemic flu, but more research is needed to assess the extent to which increased recruitment would help in other situations where the blood supply is diminished.[13]

Pathogen-related threats to the blood supply are a significant and perennial concern to FDA and blood centers. In the event of an emergent pathogen, where testing is not yet available, deferrals could significantly reduce the number of usable units of blood. The recent outbreak of the Zika virus has posed a test case for such an event. In March 2016, HHS responded to the inability to test blood for Zika from donors in Puerto Rico by facilitating the shipment of blood collected by ABC, ARC, and Blood Centers of America (BCA) centers in areas of the United States that did not have active transmission of Zika to Puerto Rico.[14]

In fact, the federal government plays an instrumental role both in helping the blood system cope with unexpected shocks, such as Zika, and in investing in the development of screening tests and PRTs to ensure the safety of the blood system. In this sense, the U.S. taxpayer already pays at least some part of the "insurance bill" required to maintain smooth operation of the U.S. blood system during shocks. SOC operates to coordinate government medical "preparedness, response and recovery efforts" in the event of public health emergencies. SOC can assist local governments with logistical support to move blood in the event of such emergencies, such as in the case of the Zika virus. Within ASPR, BARDA can also spearhead investments in innovations, such as pathogen testing and PRT. For example, BARDA is currently financing the development of a test to detect Zika. Although the government can and does serve an important role in helping the industry cope with unexpected risks and uncertainty, the ability of the government to facilitate these types of responses may lessen as excess capacity is removed from the market.

Demand-Side Shocks

Recent public health emergencies have demonstrated the agility of the blood system in responding to emergencies. The September 11, 2001, terrorist attacks resulted in an additional 258 units of blood needed, which were easily supplied by what hospitals had in storage.[15] In fact, following the surge in donations, estimated at more than 475,000 additional units immediately following the attacks, ARC had to discard approximately

---

Shocks," *PLoS One*, Vol. 6, No. 7, 2011, p. e21752; Christel Kamp, Margarethe Heiden, Olaf Henseler, and Rainer Seitz, "Management of Blood Supplies During an Influenza Pandemic," *Transfusion*, Vol. 50, No. 1, 2010, pp. 231–239.

[13]   An et al., 2011.

[14]   HHS Press Office, "HHS Ships Blood Products to Puerto Rico in Response to Zika Outbreak," press release, March 7, 2016.

[15]   P. J. Schmidt, "Blood and Disaster—Supply and Demand," *New England Journal of Medicine*, Vol. 346, No. 8, 2002, p. 617.

17 percent of donations that became outdated in October 2001,[16] and an estimated 250,000 units nationally were discarded.[17] It is also worth noting that although donations do tend to increase in the wake of a public health emergency or disaster, those units cannot be used immediately, as they require at least two days of testing and processing.[18] Mass casualty and disaster events prior to the September 11 attacks have shown similar patterns of actual blood needed and amounts donated.[19] More recently, the terrorist attacks in London's subway system in 2005 and the 2011 Japanese earthquake required 440 units[20] and 1,938 units of RBCs, respectively.[21] Although these events occurred outside the United States, it is worth noting that these public health emergencies resulted in considerably more blood demand than was needed in response to the September 11 attacks (or the previous disasters that Schmidt discusses).[22] Thus, although there appears to be little evidence of blood shortages among both the reviewed U.S. events and the international events, the range of blood units potentially needed is large.

Overall, demand-side shocks to date have resulted only in modest shifts in the amount of blood needed, and they have typically been accompanied by surges in blood donations. This does not necessarily imply that a blood system without surge capacity will be able to respond similarly. Some key stakeholders who we interviewed argued that the system's current trajectory could lead to an environment with decreased resiliency or ability of centers to respond to such emergencies.

Broader Systemwide Shocks

In addition to shocks that directly affect either the number of individuals who can donate blood or the number of individuals who need blood on any given day, there are other potential scenarios that can cause significant disruptions to the blood system by imposing logistical challenges that make it difficult for blood to be moved quickly around the country or for key medical professionals or blood establishment personnel to do their jobs.[23] For example, a catastrophic earthquake in a major U.S. city

---

[16] Schmidt, 2002.

[17] GAO, 2002.

[18] GAO, 2002.

[19] Schmidt, 2002.

[20] S. M. Glasgow, S. Allard, H. Doughty, P. Spreadborough, and E. Watkins "Blood and Bombs: The Demand and Use of Blood Following the London Bombings of 7 July 2005–A Retrospective Review," *Transfusion Medicine*, Vol. 22, No. 4, 2012, pp. 244–250.

[21] Karen Quillen and C. John Luckey, "Blood and Bombs: Blood Use After the Boston Marathon Bombing of April 15, 2013," *Transfusion*, Vol. 54, No. 4, 2014, pp. 1202–1203.

[22] Schmidt, 2002.

[23] Shimian Zou, "Potential Impact of Pandemic Influenza on Blood Safety and Availability," *Transfusion Medicine Reviews*, Vol. 20, No. 3, 2006, pp. 181–189; Ann B. Zimrin, and John R. Hess, "Planning for Pandemic

could not only damage buildings and infrastructure in the city but could also impede immediate transportation from other regions.[24] In such an event, damage within the city could affect blood centers and hospitals' current stocks of blood (loss of electricity could affect the conditions in which the blood is stored, making it unusable) and collection sites' abilities to collect, test, and process additional blood. Significant damage to roads could preclude medical providers and other personnel from being able to reach hospitals or sites of need.

Other Uncertainty and Risk in the Blood System

Another significant source of risk in the blood system is the limited shelf life of blood products—in particular, the risk of expiration. There are costs associated with the collecting, testing, and transporting of blood, regardless of whether it is ultimately used. If the expiration of blood products becomes increasingly common, more blood must be collected to meet demand for blood services. Expiration also carries disposal costs, which are significant, given that discarded blood must be treated as a potential biohazard.

In the present market, blood centers and hospitals are responsible for the risk of shortage or expiration, depending on the contractual agreements. In the event that hospitals own the blood on purchase, they bear the risk of expiration. In the consignment-type arrangements that are much more common, hospitals can hedge against shortages by ordering extra blood and only paying for used blood. Blood centers typically pay the transportation costs associated with moving unused blood to a location in these cases. Blood centers can also stipulate that units be returned prior to expiration. Whether these and any other costs associated with ensuring the availability of blood are incorporated into the price that hospitals pay for blood is an empirical question. If blood centers demand higher prices to cover these additional costs, then hospitals could be paying for some or all of the costs associated with managing these risks.

Wastage

In agreements where hospitals own the blood upon delivery, we would expect there to be some amount of wastage reflecting hospitals ordering too much blood for insurance purposes—that is, to avoid not having enough blood in the event of an emergency. However, the absence of wastage does not necessarily imply that hospitals are not incurring the cost of insurance, because, for example, hospitals and their blood center suppliers can and do distribute blood to other hospitals in the event of excess, and also because some of this insurance premium might go toward maintaining spare

---

Influenza: Effect of a Pandemic on the Supply and Demand for Blood Products in the United States," *Transfusion* Vol. 47, No. 6, 2007, pp. 1071–1079.

[24] Lucile M. Jones, Richard Bernknopf, Dale Cox, James Goltz, Kenneth Hudnut, Dennis Mileti, Suzanne Perry, Daniel Ponti, Keith Porter, and Michael Reichle, "The Shakeout Scenario," *U.S. Geological Survey Open-File Report*, California Geological Survey, Vol. 1150, No. 25, 2008.

(unused) collection and processing capacity within blood centers. The extent to which this occurs and who bears the costs associated with these transactions is unclear. While expired and unused blood sometimes can be used for research purposes, it can also result in additional costs from biohazard disposal.

In consignment-type arrangements where hospitals can return unused blood, we would expect hospitals to request more blood than needed, which would require greater logistical efforts and costs for the blood centers in aggregate. Many blood centers and hospitals we interviewed noted that although inventory management software products are used, there does not seem to be a system integrated across all hospitals and blood centers that could facilitate a more-efficient second market for the unused blood that needs to be reshelved with a second or third hospital. However, DoD does have an integrated system of inventory management used across all hospitals.

In many cases, blood transfer is decided on a daily basis, typically following a morning phone call from the hospital to the blood center. To cover this market gap, new software solutions have now been offered to hospitals and blood centers—although the use of such technology to facilitate monitoring and ordering of blood units is not universal.

Overall, there were 14,237,000 units of whole blood and apheresis RBCs collected in 2013,[25] and less than 2 percent of those units were outdated (expired before use). This is only slightly less than the 3 percent of units outdated in 2004 (see Figure 6.1).[26] In sum, the blood system in aggregate seems to have very little outdating; however, what this implies for the value of blood is less clear.

Public Preparedness and Surge Capacity

Ensuring that blood is available when needed might have a broader value to society beyond any value to hospitals. However, because hospital demand for blood is derived from patient demand for blood, we would expect a direct relationship between the hospital's value of blood and an aggregated societal value of blood. Economic theory suggests that if hospitals do not directly bear additional costs to obtain unexpected or emergency units, they might undervalue having a reliable supply of blood on hand.

Some key stakeholders have suggested that the blood supply should be thought of as a "public good." Public goods (as opposed to "private goods") are defined in economics as goods for which one person's consumption of the good does not impede another person's consumption (referred to as nonrivalrous) and which we cannot prevent others from consuming (nonexcludable); clean air, national security, and public parks are

---

[25] Chung et al., 2016.

[26] We were unable to test whether these differences are statistically different, as we did not have access to the underlying data.

Figure 6.1
Blood Units Transfused, Outdated, and Not Used, 2004 to 2013

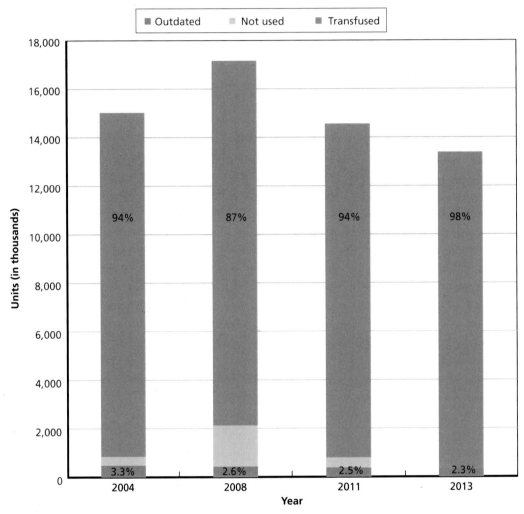

SOURCES: NBCUS, 2004–2013. The number of units not used was calculated as the difference between the total units of blood collected and the number of units either transfused or outdated. For 2013, this was not statistically different from zero.
RAND RR1575-6.2

classic examples of public goods. Although one person's consumption of blood does prevent another from using that same unit of blood, and we can prevent others from consuming that same unit, one could argue that the critical infrastructure for blood is a public good, similar to our water or electricity infrastructure. Without a surge capacity to meet emergency needs, the blood system faces a classic free-rider problem in which the cost of a common resource is not distributed equally. In this case, the surge capacity is akin to a public good and we end up with a kind of "market failure," specifically that the quantity demanded does not meet the quantity supplied in the market and a more-efficient allocation could be achieved. In this case, the blood system might not provide an adequate surge capacity on its own. Typical economic solutions to such public goods problems involve either the government stepping in to incentivize private investment in maintaining a surge capacity of blood for disasters or the government providing the infrastructure itself.

There are many examples of government interventions to provide public goods related to public health and preparedness—for example, the National Pharmaceutical Stockpile for use in responding to bioterrorism events, HRSA grants to provide primary care to underserved populations, and CDC surveillance programs.

There are also analogous government interventions in water and electricity that could provide lessons to the blood industry. First, much of the monopoly created through government intervention in the water and electricity supplies is directly related to the economies of scale in the production of each of these economies. There are large investments that need to be made to efficiently produce electricity and clean water. The incremental cost of production is relatively small in both of these sectors. As such, as production increases, the average cost of production falls, and it makes economic and social sense to have a single operator so that prices for individual consumers are as low as possible, and there are not wasted, redundant investments if more than one firm tries to serve an area. Because of these types of economies of scale, public utility commissions have been established so that there is a provider even in unprofitable areas and to set a rate of return on investment, and in turn a price, so that firms want to invest in an area. These public utility commissions also determine the service area for the industry so that there is not competition among firms to provide the same product. These are commonly referred to in economics as *natural monopolies*. Additionally, the electricity sector is mandated to have 99.9 percent reliability, which means that it must have excess capacity for generation to meet peak demand that typically occurs during summer afternoons when air conditioning use is highest. This is similar in some respects to having sufficient blood supplies to meet large-scale disasters, but the marginal cost of obtaining a given unit of blood is likely to be nonlinear. That is, getting the initial blood donation in a given market is likely to be easier (and less costly) than getting the last person in a market to donate blood. Thus, marginal recruitment costs likely decrease initially but then will begin to increase as more individuals donate blood (because then there are fewer individuals who have not yet been recruited).

The federal government also subsidizes infrastructure improvements for drinking water in some communities. These subsidies are generally for the water and wastewater treatment facilities that communities require to meet drinking water standards, defraying some of the high cost of initial investment in water and wastewater treatment facilities. Because there are a large number of small communities geographically dispersed, it does not make sense to make even larger investments in the distribution system. Instead, it is preferable to have a series of large investments in small and rural communities.

There are two main concerns within the public utilities that can be directly related to maintaining a surge capacity of blood. First, there are potentially large investments in facilities for the storage and gathering of blood for the purposes of maintaining a surge capacity for emergencies. However, the federal government could harness already-established private facilities and provide subsidies for regional storage of excess blood for emergency use. Because blood has a short shelf life, maintenance and variable costs could be significant. We would first need an estimate of what constitutes an adequate surge capacity to assess the feasibility of these approaches.

A second related issue is how emergency blood would be distributed in various scenarios to address surge capacity concerns. In the case of electricity, the distribution network is large, forming a grid over the entire country. A federal mandate requires that electricity companies must provide electricity to all households, not exclusively to urban households with lower distribution costs. This is why the U.S. electricity system supports a small number of large producers and a large distribution network. In the case of water, there is a large number of facilities with a relatively small distribution network centered on each water treatment facility. For rural households, water is provided by individual wells, with very little treatment by the household. How the blood system would utilize existing blood center and hospital networks to address emergency demands is unclear. Again, to consider how the government might intervene to help provide the surge capacity as a public good, we would need a better understanding of the costs of the current system of distribution.

Conclusions

In this chapter, we drew on economic theory to consider how the blood system currently addresses uncertainty and the extent to which there might be alternative approaches. We described the current cost structures and estimates of the market equilibrium price of blood. Although we were not able to ascertain whether that price already includes an insurance value or what the reservation price of patients and hospitals is, we examined previous studies about how the market has historically responded to exogenous shocks to both the supply of and demand for blood, which might help us to empirically observe whether the market already supports (i.e., already pays for the insurance of) excess capacity to meet surges in demand or declines in supply. Finally, we considered blood as a public good and discussed how government intervention might help maintain a surge capacity of blood for disaster preparedness. In our review of how the market has responded to exogenous shocks in the quantity of blood supplied or demanded, we generally found that the market has historically been capable of responding to those shocks without severe systemwide repercussions, indicating that some combination of blood center, hospital, and U.S. government resources has already paid for some degree of insurance protection. However, we note that most past investments in excess capacity might have been the unintentional result of centers' slow response to the decrease in the demand for blood, and that there might be other shocks with broader effects, such as an earthquake, that yield less-fortunate results. Moreover, as the overall blood market continues to shrink, the agility of these players to respond might be diminished. A key research question currently beyond the scope of this report will be a study quantifying the excess capacity required to meet various shocks under various scenarios and forecasting the costs involved in maintaining blood system surge capacity that could meet demand for blood under these scenarios.

In summary, the insurance value of blood is a useful concept for quantifying the risks and uncertainty that both hospitals and society face. In practice, it is unclear whether the equilibrium market price that we observe in the blood market already incorporates that value, and, if so, who is paying for it. Members of society also clearly value having a robust and safe blood supply, and although we can crudely approximate that value, the policy implications are less clear. The federal government currently plays a role in serving to buffer large systemwide shocks that might occur. This, coupled with the empirical evidence that the market has not suffered large shortages or had significant negative patient outcomes, makes it difficult to suggest that further government intervention is needed to maintain emergency surge capacity. More research is needed to determine whether larger catastrophes might overwhelm the surge capacity of the U.S. blood system or whether patients could be at risk.

CHAPTER SEVEN

Emergency Preparedness Risk Assessment

Introduction

Public health emergencies and mass casualty events are uncommon and unpredictable incidences that can result in high civilian morbidity and mortality and overwhelm local health care systems. Emergent situations could disrupt the U.S. blood system in two main ways: (1) Disasters could cause a surge in demand for blood caused by mass trauma, for example, in the acute aftermath of an earthquake or the bombing of a building, or (2) there could be a reduction in supply caused by the lack of available donors in the event of a radiological attack or global pandemic. In mass trauma settings, hemorrhage is the leading cause of preventable mortality, accounting for almost 50 percent of deaths in the first 24 hours.[1] Resuscitation of patients suffering from hemorrhage involves high ratios of blood components, such as fresh or frozen plasma, platelets, and RBCs. As such, there is a surge in the immediate demand for blood products. This is further exacerbated by the fact that blood must be type-matched to individual patients, and shortages of rare blood types and products can hamper recovery efforts. Therefore, the timely availability and appropriate delivery of the range of blood products is essential to improve survival in severely injured patients. Conversely, when healthy donors who are eligible to donate blood are in short supply, the challenge to blood centers is in managing routine demand (as opposed to surge capacity) for blood products in the absence of a normal supply.

As blood is a critical input into many health care services, the blood system must cope with day-to-day variation in supply and demand and respond to surges in demand caused by a wide variety of potential emergent situations. This chapter focuses on the resiliency of the blood supply to several disaster scenarios that would either cause a massive reduction in potential donors (blood supply) or require surge capacity on the part of the U.S. blood system. We describe the various components, players, complexities, and decision points in the blood supply chain, followed by an analysis of the effect

---

[1] Justin Sobrino and Shahid Shafi, "Timing and Causes of Death After Injuries," *Proceedings (Baylor University Medical Center)*, Vol. 26, No. 2, 2013, p. 120.

of various disaster scenarios on the blood system based on literature from past emergencies, where available and applicable.

Methodology

Blood Supply Chain Influence Diagrams

Risk evaluation of the blood supply chain first requires knowledge of the various players, components, and decision points in the complex system. Based on the blood supply chain literature and expert interviews with individual blood centers, ARC, hospitals, and product vendors, we outlined the major players in the blood supply chain and identified key influencers and decision points, or "nodes," in the system. Such nodes, representing individual variables on which the supply chain is dependent, are outlined in influence diagrams. Influence diagrams illustrate the critical activities that occur between donor to recipient and the main factors that influence such activities, providing a framework to assess the potential disruptions to the supply chain caused by various emergent situations. We restricted this analysis to the tangible aspects (people, activities, and supplies) of the supply chain, as regulations and financial considerations are discussed elsewhere in this report.

Case Studies or Scenarios

Each segment of the blood supply chain faces a wide range of emergency risks with differing levels of potential impact, both with respect to the likelihood of the emergency occurring and with respect to the magnitude of the effect, should the emergency occur. In order to categorize risk factors, we began with a list of likely emergencies identified in the national planning scenarios and by ARC,[2] which include weather-related emergencies (drought, earthquake, flood, heat wave, hurricane), other natural disasters (wildfire, volcano), disease and health-related emergencies (flu, poisoning, food safety), terrorism, and infrastructure emergencies (highway, power outage, IT). The most probable risks to the blood supply tend to threaten multiple nodes in the blood supply chain.

We narrowed this list of possible emergency disruptions to the blood supply by categorizing events across two key dimensions: (1) the probability of the scenario occurring, and (2) the estimated magnitude or size of the consequence (the impact on the blood system). We differentiated between low- and high-likelihood events (the vertical axis in Figure 7.1) and low- and high-impact events (the horizontal axis in Figure 7.1). We note that the probability of a weather-related emergency or natural disaster affecting the blood supply can range from low to high, as some events might have little or no

---

2   ARC, "Types of Emergencies," undated-c; Homeland Security Council, "National Planning Scenarios: Executive Summaries," Version 20.2, Washington, D.C.: U.S. Department of Homeland Security, 2006a.

Figure 7.1
Categorizing Risk Factors Facing the Blood Supply

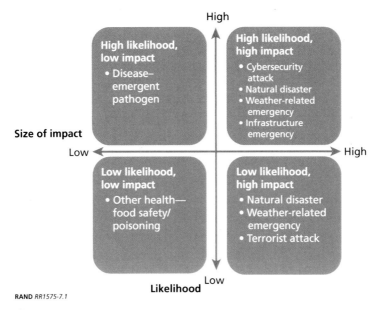

impact on the blood supply (e.g., drought), but others can have catastrophic outcomes that could affect several nodes in the supply chain (e.g., hurricane or earthquake).

Secondly, we assessed whether each emergent situation represented an acute or rapid onset disaster, such as a terrorist attack or an earthquake, or a more gradual and sustained event, such as a drought or a flood. Finally, we considered whether a disaster represented a shock to the demand side or the supply side of the blood system.[3] Combining these factors, we defined three emergency scenarios that span the range of probabilities, effects, and acuity: (1) a natural disaster, (2) a terrorist attack, and (3) a global pandemic. The characteristics of these events are summarized in Table 7.1.

The three scenarios represent a range of likelihoods, effects, and demand-side or supply-side shocks. In choosing these emergencies, we reviewed the literature to ascertain the probability of these emergencies occurring and estimates of their impact on the blood system or their broad impacts if specific estimates of impacts on the blood system were not available. In Chapter Six, we discussed how the market price and quantity might shift in response to such shocks, but in this chapter we focus on how such shocks might affect nodes in the supply chain.

Scenario 1: A Local Natural Disaster

For catastrophic natural disasters, the probability is variable; however, the probability of an earthquake or hurricane in some large metropolitan areas (e.g., San Francisco, Cali-

---

[3] For simplicity and scope, we ruled out disaster scenarios that have a minimal impact on the supply chain, such as a drought.

Table 7.1
Disaster Scenario Characteristics

	Onset	Likelihood	Effect	Shock to Supply or Demand
Scenario 1: Natural disaster	Acute or sustained	Low to high	Low to high	Both
Scenario 2: Terrorist attack	Acute	Low	High	Both
Scenario 3: Pandemic	Sustained	High	Low	Supply only

fornia, or New Orleans, Louisiana) is relatively high. For example, there is a 63-percent chance of an earthquake hitting the San Francisco Bay Area in the next 30 years.[4] The effects of these types of natural disasters can be significant: The Shakeout Scenario study,[5] a simulation of the effects of a large earthquake in San Francisco, suggests as many as 750 trauma injuries; $113 billion in property damage, including buildings and roads; and another $100 billion in business interruptions and traffic delay costs. Finding enough blood for 750 trauma injuries might not be the biggest challenge, if, for example, each patient needed 20 units of blood (which is considerably more than the six units needed by the median trauma patient), as that would require 15,000 units of blood, which could conceivably be gathered within the first 24 hours following the earthquake.[6] What is less certain (and potentially more of a challenge) would be the ability to transport blood, even locally within the Bay Area, if there were extensive damages to infrastructure that impeded transportation. Thus, the magnitude of such an event could be substantial.

Scenario 2: A Local Disaster Involving a Terrorist Attack

Although the odds of a terrorist attack are low, the effects could be extensive, depending on where it occurred and the extent to which the area was prepared. Historically, terrorist attacks in the United States have not resulted in large increases in the demand for blood, but they could impose significant damage to infrastructure, affecting multiple nodes in the blood supply chain.[7]

Scenario 3: A Global Pandemic

The probability of an influenza pandemic or other emergent pathogen affecting the blood supply (through increased deferrals, for example) varies. There are seasonal

---

[4]   U.S. Geological Survey, "2008 Bay Area Earthquake Probabilities," last revised June 30, 2016.

[5]   Jones et al., 2008.

[6]   J. J. Como, R. P. Dutton, T. M. Scalea, B. B. Edelman, J. R. Hess, "Blood Transfusion Rates in the Care of Acute Trauma," *Transfusion*, Vol. 44, No. 6, 2004, pp. 809–813.

[7]   Schmidt, 2002.

surges, for example, in cases of influenza. Influenza pandemics are, by definition, more difficult to predict, as they occur when influenza spreads beyond the usual seasonal scale, and they occur irregularly. In the 20th century, there were three influenza pandemics affecting nearly 30 percent of the world population.[8] Experts warn that emerging disease pandemics—for new strains of influenza or emergent pathogens, such as the Zika virus—are increasingly likely, as international travel has increased. Parts of the United States are already facing the spread of the Zika virus, and, until a test is developed to detect its presence in blood, there is likely to be a large number of deferrals (like in Puerto Rico).

Risk Assessment

We reviewed the evidence from recent disasters published in peer-reviewed literature, as well as in the news media, to assess the resilience of the blood supply chain in the three disaster scenarios outlined. For Scenario 1, humanitarian activities in the aftermath of Hurricane Katrina in 2005 and Hurricane Sandy in 2012 provided illustrations of the range of impacts of a local natural disaster. The June 2016 shootings in Orlando, Florida; the terrorist attacks of September 11, 2001, in New York City; and the 1995 Oklahoma City bombing provided evidence for Scenario 2. For Scenario 3, while there are not many recent examples of pandemics resulting in mass casualties in the United States, lessons learned from the previous two scenarios, the ongoing Zika crisis, and estimates of personnel losses from global flu pandemics helped inform our conclusions.

Based on existing evidence where available, we assessed the vulnerability of each node in the blood supply chain to potential future threats with directional low, medium, and high scores across four main domains: (1) the magnitude of the expected impact on the particular health care market or geographic area, (2) the local node vulnerability that reflects how the blood supply chain node is impacted in the immediate vicinity of the emergent situation (i.e., the New York City blood centers in the aftermath of the September 11 attacks), (3) the overall risk of the threat for that particular node nationwide (i.e., all blood centers after the September 11 attacks), and (4) the ability of the national system to absorb or redistribute blood and blood supplies quickly to address a local event. In addition, we assessed the potential of the national blood system as a whole to absorb or mitigate supply or demand shocks with a simple qualitative score. The ultimate risk score for each node is dependent on these two factors, along with the magnitude of the impact of the disaster scenario.

---

[8] Homeland Security Council, *National Strategy for Pandemic Influenza: Implementation Plan*, Washington, D.C.: U.S. Department of Homeland Security, 2006b.

Blood Supply Chain and Risk Assessment

We briefly review the blood supply chain in the United States, as described in Chapter Two, which is a complex system (see Figure 7.2). In our risk assessment analysis, we focused on two main nodes in the blood supply chain: donors and blood centers.

Several features of the U.S. blood system make it challenging from a strategic planning standpoint:

- Blood is a perishable commodity, and each component of blood has a different acceptable shelf life.
- The supply of eligible and willing donors is irregular: Blood is drawn from a widely variable number of people at differing times and locations. Additionally, seasonal flu patterns, trends in global travel, emerging infectious diseases, and weather can all affect the supply of donors and disease-free blood.

Figure 7.2
Blood Supply Chain

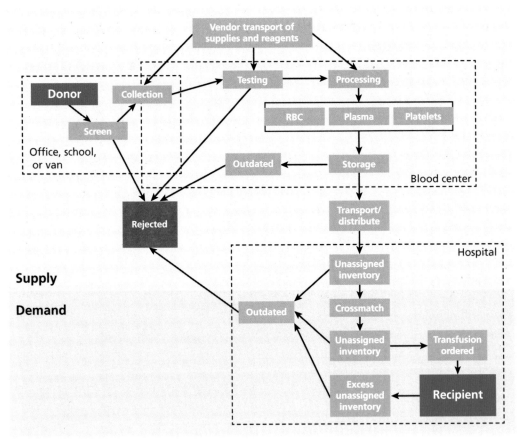

- The demand for blood and blood products is also uncertain: While the number of elective surgeries, oncology patients, and blood disorder patients requiring blood may be relatively predictable day to day, trauma and obstetrics demands for blood can be more difficult to predict, especially for outlier patients requiring many units.
- Donor and recipient blood types must be cross-matched, creating further complexity in meeting supply and demand.
- Unpredictable events, such as global pandemics, natural disasters, and terrorist activities, can impact both supply and demand of blood products. In the end, the goal of the system is to produce an adequate safe supply that meets fluctuations in demand without dramatic shortages while minimizing outdates and waste.[9]

Donors

In the United States, approximately 14.2 million units of whole blood were collected in 2013 from approximately 12. 8 million volunteer donors.[10] Estimates suggest that 3 percent to 5 percent of the U.S. population donates an average of approximately 1.5 times per year.[11] Such numbers can be used to illustrate two key things about the general population's attitude about blood donation: (1) A very large proportion of potentially eligible donors do not actively donate blood; and (2) it is difficult to maintain a donor pool, particularly in light of the regular addition of new deferral or temporary rejection criteria aimed at improving safety.

A large body of research has been conducted on the motivations and barriers to donation.[12] Positive influences on blood donation include an intrinsic sense of duty and altruism, empathy, perceived societal need for blood products, experience with a friend

---

[9] Jeroen Beliën and Hein Forcé, "Supply Chain Management of Blood Products: A Literature Review," *European Journal of Operational Research*, Vol. 217, No. 1, 2012, pp. 116.

[10] Chung et al., 2016.

[11] HHS, 2011a; Richard J. Davey, "Recruiting Blood Donors: Challenges and Opportunities," *Transfusion*, Vol. 44, No. 4, 2004, pp. 597–600.

[12] Theresa W. Gillespie and Christopher D. Hillyer, "Blood Donors and Factors Impacting the Blood Donation Decision," *Transfusion Medicine Reviews*, Vol. 16, No. 2, 2002, pp. 115–130; John T. Cacioppo and Wendi L. Gardner, "What Underlies Medical Donor Attitudes and Behavior?" *Health Psychology*, Vol. 12, No. 4, 1993, p. 269; Eamonn Ferguson and Peter A. Bibby, "Predicting Future Blood Donor Returns: Past Behavior, Intentions, and Observer Effects," *Health Psychology*, Vol. 21, No. 5, 2002, p. 513; Dorothy D. Nguyen, Deborah A. DeVita, Nora V. Hirschler, and Edward L. Murphy, "Blood Donor Satisfaction and Intention of Future Donation," *Transfusion*, Vol. 48, No. 4, 2008, pp. 742–748; Eamonn Ferguson, Christopher R. France, Charles Abraham, Blaine Ditto, and Paschal Sheeran "Improving Blood Donor Recruitment and Retention: Integrating Theoretical Advances from Social and Behavioral Science Research Agendas," *Transfusion*, Vol. 47, No. 11, 2007, pp. 1999–2010.; K. P. H. Lemmens,C. Abraham, T. Hoekstra, R.A.C. Ruiter, W. L. A. M. De Kort, J. Brug, and H. P. Schaalma "Why Don't Young People Volunteer to Give Blood? An Investigation of the Correlates of Donation Intentions Among Young Nondonors," *Transfusion*, Vol. 45, No. 6, 2005, pp. 945–955; Christopher R. France, Janis L. France, Marios Roussos, and Blaine Ditto "Mild Reactions to Blood Donation Predict a Decreased Likelihood of Donor Return," *Transfusion and Apheresis Science*, Vol. 30, No.1, 2004, pp. 17–22.

or loved one who had needed blood at some time in the past, such as social pressures, the influence of friends and family, positive experiences associated with donation, and improving self-worth.[13] Negative influences include deferral upon screening (for any of the multiple deferral criteria), inconvenience, wait time, staff unfriendliness, negative reactions (fainting or light-headedness), and fear (of needles, blood, pain, or disease discovery).[14] Additionally, evidence suggests that some deferrals, such as those among individuals with a higher risk of donating blood containing blood-borne pathogens and those with low hemoglobin counts, will also make those individuals less likely to donate in the future.[15] Combining findings from this research with our own expert interviews, we developed an influence diagram[16] illustrating key factors that influence a particular individual's decision to donate blood (Figure 7.3). Green ovals represent decisions that can be influenced by emergent situations. For example, donors may be more motivated to donate when they see a large casualty toll from a terrorist attack and may perceive greater need.

In general, donor shortages in regional disasters, such as small-scale terrorist attacks and natural disasters, can be counteracted by increased donor activity elsewhere, which would require some mechanism to redistribute blood. The blood system currently utilizes exchanges systems where blood centers sell extra units to other blood centers, which could be used in such cases. Additionally, SOC can also help shift blood quickly in cases of emergency. However, in the case of true mass casualty events, such as a global flu pandemic or a large radiological detonation, the donor supply may be critically compromised, and blood centers may be unable to meet routine and emergent demands in blood. As such, donor outreach and communication regarding acute demand are critical to managing the blood supply chain during disasters. There may also be cases with weather-related or natural disasters where blood can be flown in from another part of the country but cannot be quickly deployed to sites of need (e.g., in cases where roads or infrastructure are inoperable).

Donors' Activities During Natural Disasters
A natural disaster can have an effect on donor behavior in a few notable ways, including

- Concerns for personal safety in the aftermath of a disaster (e.g., downed power lines, felled trees) may lead to cancellation of donation appointments or, on wider scales, of office- or school-based blood drives.

---

[13]   Gillespie and Hillyer, 2002; Cacioppo and Gardner, 1993; Ferguson and Bibby, 2002; Nguyen et al., 2008.

[14]   Nguyen et al., 2008.

[15]   Brian Custer, Artina Chinn, Nora V. Hirschler, Michael P. Busch, and Edward L. Murphy, "The Consequences of Temporary Deferral on Future Whole Blood Donation," *Transfusion*, Vol. 47, No. 8, 2007, pp. 1514–1523.

[16]   Influence diagrams are a graphical representation of key elements of decisionmaking. Each oval represents a decisionmaking factor, and each line represents the activity that the decisionmaking affects.

Figure 7.3
Key Donor Influences and Decision Nodes

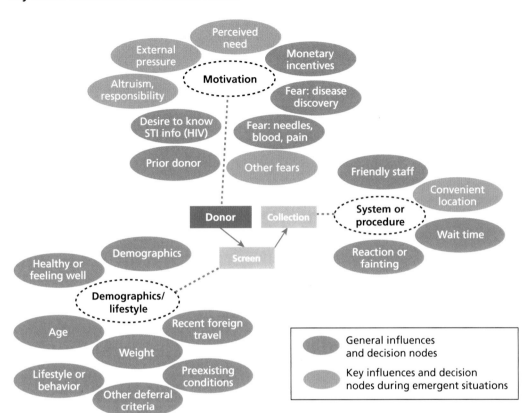

RAND *RR1575-7.3*

NOTE: STI = sexually transmitted infection.

- Caregiving time of friends and family members affected by the disaster may lead to fewer donations.
- Imposed restrictions to free movement such as police barriers and border closures, during acute situations may hamper donations.
- Catastrophes and mass casualties often bring out a sense of altruism in people who have not been affected, leading to a surge in donors.

Historically, there is demonstrable evidence of a decrease in donor activities in the immediate impact area of a natural disaster and a surge of blood donations elsewhere in the country. For example, in the immediate aftermath of Hurricane Katrina, massive infrastructure barriers prevented donors from attending blood drives in New Orleans.[17] However, donations elsewhere in the country in response to the disaster led

---

17 Meg Farris, "Critical Shortage: Blood Center Down to 1-Day Supply," WWL-TV, June 10, 2016.

to an increase in the national blood supply.[18] Similarly, Hurricane Sandy led to significant reductions in local donations, estimated at approximately 10,000 units.[19] However, altruistic donors elsewhere in the country helped in the recovery effort. Outside the United States, similar trends have been noticed after the earthquakes in Japan, China, and Chile.[20] Therefore, surpluses in supply in unaffected regions can be transported to the affected blood centers in the vicinity of disaster zones to mitigate local shortages.

Donors' Activities During Terrorist Attacks

The donor response to terrorist attacks is very similar to that of a natural disaster: There is a surge in donor activity in unaffected areas. Perhaps the most well-documented incidence of a donor surge occurred in the immediate aftermath of the September 11 attacks. It is estimated that blood centers across the country collected more than 475,000 additional units immediately following the attacks.[21] Similarly, following the Boston marathon bombing, marathoners and spectators alike lined up to donate blood, so much so that Massachusetts General Hospital and the Red Cross stopped accepting donations by mid-afternoon on the day of the attack.[22] More recently, blood centers worldwide saw an uptick in donations in the immediate aftermath of the bombings in Paris and Belgium, as well as the recent shooting events in San Bernardino, California, and Orlando, Florida.[23] The uptick in donations in times of emergencies, however, cannot be used immediately and, as discussed in Chapter Six, in some cases actually results in more wastage.

Donors' Activities During Pandemics

The influence of a large-scale pandemic on the blood supply is largely a theoretical exercise, as, thankfully, there has not been recent historic evidence of large-scale, mass-casualty illnesses in the United States. However, projections based on the pandemic of 1918, in which 675,000 people died in the United States and 50 million worldwide,

---

[18] Kumudu K. S. Kuruppu, "Management of Blood System in Disasters," *Biologicals*, Vol. 38, No.1, 2010, pp. 87–90.

[19] ARC, "Sandy Forces Cancellation of About 300 Blood Drives," October 30, 2012.

[20] An et al., 2011; Kamp et al., 2010.

[21] Carl H. Schultz, Kristi L. Koenig, and Eric K. Noji, "A Medical Disaster Response to Reduce Immediate Mortality After an Earthquake," *New England Journal of Medicine*, Vol. 334, No. 7, 1996, pp. 438–444; Schmidt, 2002; GAO, 2002.

[22] Nina Strochlic, "Boston Marathon Explosions: The Heroes Who Responded to the Blasts," *The Daily Beast*, April 16, 2013.

[23] Rick Neale, "Blood Donations Skyrocket in Florida After Orlando Massacre," Florida Today, KHOU, June 30, 2016; Anas Khan, "Level of Willingness to Report to Work During a Pandemic Among the Emergency Department Health Care Professionals," *Asian Journal of Medical Sciences* Vol. 5, No. 3, 2014, pp. 58–62.

suggest that 30 percent to 50 percent of the population could be infected or disabled.[24] As such, it is generally believed that a mass disease outbreak will significantly limit the number of healthy donors.[25] One recent study has identified 86 emerging (or recently emerged) pathogens that threaten the safety of the blood supply, which suggests the need to plan for management of transfusion-transmitted infections but, more importantly, also the need for an investigation of prevalence in the donor populations, with an eye toward developing interventions and screening.[26] Additionally, donors may not perceive the need to donate following a pandemic in the same way that they would after a weather emergency or terrorist attack. As such, pandemics will have three main deterrent effects to donors:

1. Concerns for personal safety may lead to cancellation of donation appointments or, on wider scales, of office- or school-based blood drives.
2. Caregiving time of friends and family members affected by the disaster may additionally lead to fewer donations.
3. Restrictions (both external and self-imposed) to free movement during pandemic situations may additionally hamper donations.

This was demonstrated during the 2009 swine flu outbreak, which saw a 27-percent overall reduction in donations because of the cancellation of office- and school-based blood drives.[27] The nature of pandemic spreading leads to more-rapid and higher impact in large cosmopolitan centers; rural locations may be isolated from the brunt of a disease epidemic. Therefore, while a global pandemic may have a high overall impact to the donor pool as a whole, local communities may still have unaffected individuals. Overall, however, shortages in healthy donors are of particular concern during global pandemics, as the supply may be unable to meet routine demand, let alone surges in demand.

Donor Risk Assessment

Based on the available evidence, we assigned an overall risk score based on the vulnerability of donors to each disaster scenario (Table 7.2). For natural disasters and terrorist attacks, the vulnerability of local donors is a function of the magnitude of the impact (and geographic area) of the disaster at a local level. For example, a Category 2 or 3

---

[24] John G. Bartlett, "Planning for Avian Influenza," *Annals of Internal Medicine*, Vol. 145, No. 2, 2006, pp. 141–144; Zimrin and Hess, 2007.

[25] WHO, Regional Office for South-East Asia, "Pandemic H1N1 2009," New Delhi, India: WHO, 2009.

[26] Susan Stramer, F. Blaine Hollinger, Louis M. Katz, Steven Kleinman, Peyton S. Metzel, Kay R. Gregory, and Roger Y. Dodd, "Emerging Infectious Disease Agents and Their Potential Threat to Transfusion Safety," *Transfusion*, Vol. 49, No. S2, 2009, pp. 1S–29S.

[27] AABB, Interorganizational Task Force on Pandemic Influenza and the Blood Supply, Pandemic Influenza Planning, Version 2.0, Bethesda, Md., October 2009.

Table 7.2
Donor Risk Assessment Summary

	Magnitude of Impact	Local Donor Vulnerability	Overall U.S. Donor Vulnerability	National System Absorption Capacity	Overall Risk Score for Blood System
Scenario 1: Natural disaster	Low	Low	Low	High	Low
	Medium	Medium	Low	High	Low
	High	High	Low	High	Medium
Scenario 2: Terrorist attack	High	Medium	Low	High	Low
Scenario 3: Global pandemic	Low	Medium	High	Low	High

hurricane will have a low impact on the local population, mostly from coastal flooding and downed power lines. A Category 5 hurricane, however, could incapacitate the population of a coastal city, as was demonstrated during Hurricane Katrina. The impact of terrorist attacks may be similarly limited—the Orlando shooting was contained in a nightclub, leaving the majority of the Orlando population unaffected and free to donate blood. Even during the September 11 attacks, the largest terrorist attacks in the United States, the majority of the New York City population was unaffected. Additionally, during both natural disasters and terrorist attacks, donors in other, unaffected regions of the country are not at risk, and so the absorption capacity of the national blood system is high. Therefore, the overall risk score is low to medium.

For pandemics, on the other hand, local donors in certain regions may be shielded from the disease, especially in rural areas, where exposure is low. However, the overall vulnerability of donors across the country is high, and the system may not able to be able to absorb shortages over the long run. Therefore, the overall risk that a pandemic poses to the donor pool is high.

Blood Centers

Blood centers aim to ensure that enough healthy donors are recruited to maintain a safe and disease-free supply of blood that matches the hospital or patient demand for blood. Based on an analysis of the literature, supplemented by interviews with hospitals and blood centers, we developed an influence diagram summarizing the major influences and decision points related to the blood center's role in the supply chain (Figure 7.4). Major decision points and nodes are discussed next.

Figure 7.4
Key Blood Center Influences and Decision Nodes

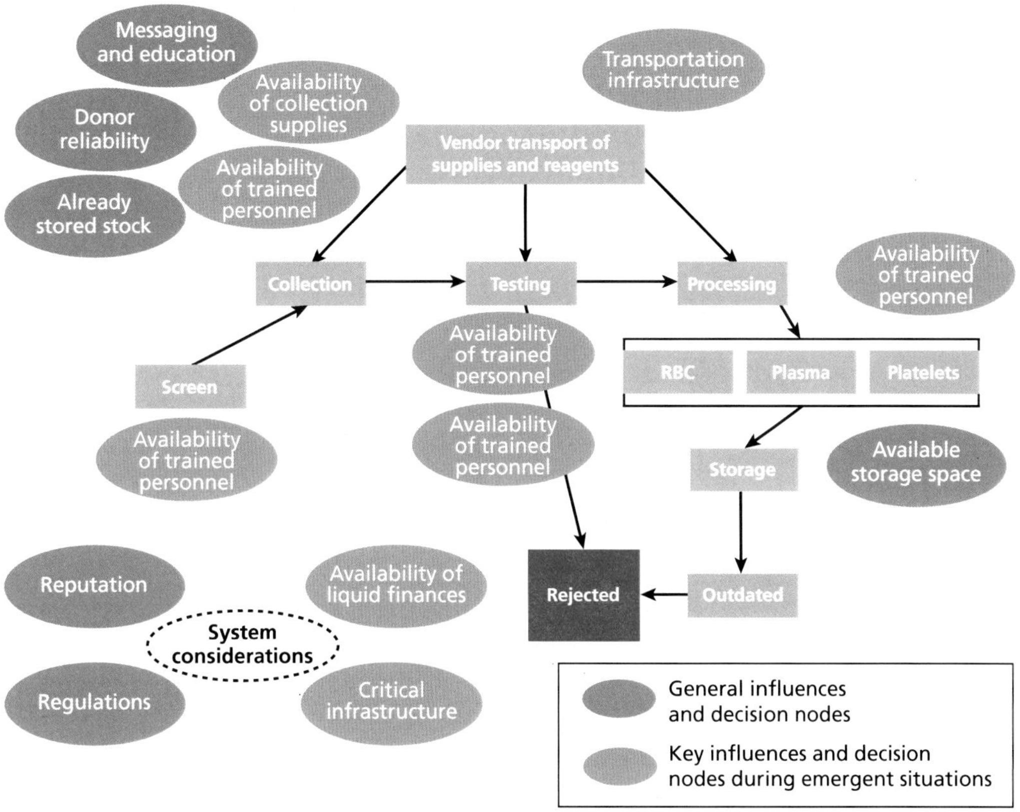

Reserve Stocks at Local Blood Centers

Blood centers must forecast demand of various blood products to anticipate routine demand. The perceived demand then influences collection of whole blood versus platelets via apheresis, as well as further fractionation of whole blood into RBCs, plasma, and platelets. Current disaster planning guidance at ARC and AABB recommends that blood centers carry at least a three-day supply of blood to meet any unexpected surges in demand. In disaster scenarios, prior to any calls for increased donation, a blood center must assess whether the current stock on hand is adequate to meet demand. Because processing and testing of blood can take up to 48 hours and typically occur outside of the blood centers, surges in demand must be met by current inventory or will require rapid movement of blood from blood collection centers to testing or processing entities, which may be difficult in times of emergency.

However, it is important to note that the consumption of reserve stocks might also lead to long-term shortages when blood centers are not able to replace supply quickly.

As such, blood centers must often buy blood from other centers that might have surplus supply and must ramp up donor recruitment. HHS can help facilitate these exchanges more quickly in emergencies and help with transportation to the extent that infrastructure is not compromised. The recovery period, during which blood centers work on restocking supply, is the most critical time for blood centers.[28]

Reserve Stocks During Natural Disasters

ABC's blood statistics data did not highlight blood centers with critical shortages immediately following Hurricanes Sandy or Katrina,[29] suggesting that blood centers were likely able to meet demand in the acute aftermath of Sandy. However, there were many calls for blood drives in the long-term aftermath of Hurricanes Katrina and Sandy to recover depleted reserves.[30]

Reserve Stocks During Terrorist Attacks

Historically, the supply at local blood centers has been sufficient to cover the immediate demand after terrorist attacks. After the Oklahoma City bombing, the local blood center director noted,

> Within moments we learned of an explosion and, recognizing that the victims would need blood, we began moving blood to the major hospitals in Oklahoma City before any of the victims had been pulled from the blast site. As it turned out, all of the emergency blood needs were met by blood that had been donated before the tragedy and was available on our shelves.[31]

Similarly, New York City hospitals did not experience shortages of blood in the immediate aftermath of the September 11 attacks.[32] After the 2016 shootings in Orlando, the Orlando blood center was able to meet acute demand. However, their activities depleted their reserve stocks, inciting donor recruitment activities to meet routine demand following the attack.[33]

---

[28] Glasgow et al., 2013; Eliat Shinar, Vered Yahalom, and Barbara G. Silverman, "Meeting Blood Requirements Following Terrorist Attacks: The Israeli Experience," *Current Opinion in Hematology*, Vol. 13, No. 6, 2006, pp. 452–456.

[29] ABC, "Stoplight Report," undated-a.

[30] David Crary, "After Superstorm Sandy Surge, Donations to Red Cross Drop," *Athens Banner-Herald*, October 29, 2015.

[31] Gilcher, 2001.

[32] Kristen Kidder, "Donor Surge: The Challenge of Managing Blood Donations During Disaster," Federal Emergency Management Agency, May 13, 2010.

[33] Paul Brinkmann, "How Blood Banks Handled Pulse Shooting, 28,000 Donors," *Orlando Sentinel*, July 1, 2016.

Reserve Stocks During Pandemics

Previous studies have predicted and used simulation modeling to estimate the impacts of a pandemic on blood reserve stocks and have suggested that emergency preparedness for pandemics should consider and plan for depletions in long-term reserve stocks at blood centers.[34] One recent example has been in observing how the system has responded to the current threat of the Zika virus. At the time of publication of this report (November 2016), the FDA had not approved an assay to detect Zika in donated blood, so screening and deferral were necessary to ensure a safe supply.[35] However, globalization is increasing travel between the United States and endemic countries, and, as such, a significant portion of potential donors are being screened out. Therefore, the United States is experiencing shortages in blood nationwide.[36] Additionally, U.S. regions and territories with high rates of Zika infection, such as Puerto Rico, are no longer collecting blood in their own populations out of fears for Zika contamination— roughly 2,500 units of blood are shipped to Puerto Rico on a weekly basis to ensure a safe blood supply.[37]

Reserve Stock Risk Assessment

Based on evidence reviewed, we summarize the risk posed to a blood system's reserve stocks in Table 7.3. During natural disasters and terrorist attacks, reserve stocks are deployed to meet surges in demand to the extent that infrastructure is still intact. Assuming that a blood center's recruitment efforts prior to the disaster result in the recommended three-day supply at any given time, the overall vulnerability of the short-term reserves is low to medium, depending on the effects and geographic scope of the disaster.

The long-term reserve vulnerability is a direct function of blood-product consumption during the acute phase of the disaster. If not many units of blood are used initially, then the long-term vulnerability is low, whereas if acute consumption is high, the long-term vulnerability is high. In addition, the national system has a relatively high capacity to compensate for a surge in local consumption during a disaster. Therefore, for natural disasters and terrorist attacks, the overall risk of the blood reserves is low to medium.

For a pandemic, on the other hand, when the pandemic has not peaked, the short-term vulnerability of blood reserves is low. However, as time passes and more

---

[34] Kamp et al., 2010; Zou, 2006; Zimrin and Hess, 2007.

[35] Didier Musso, Susan L. Stramer, and Michael P. Busch, "Zika Virus: A New Challenge for Blood Transfusion," *The Lancet*, Vol. 387, No. 10032, pp. 1993–1994.

[36] Sammy Caiola, "Blood Banks Face 'Unprecedented' Shortage Due in Part to Zika Restrictions," *Sacramento Bee*, July 5, 2016; "New York Blood Center in Short Supply, in Need of Donations," CBS New York, June 15, 2016; Rina Nakano, "Blood Banks Cite Zika Virus as Reason for Shortage," Fox 40 Sacramento, July 8, 2016.

[37] Toni Clarke, "Zika-Hit Puerto Rico Prepares to Import All of Its Blood Supplies," Reuters, February 19, 2016.

Table 7.3
Risk Assessment of Local Supply Reserves

	Magnitude of Impact	Short-Term Reserve Vulnerability	Long-Term Reserve Vulnerability	National System Absorption Capacity	Overall Risk Score for Blood System
Scenario 1: Natural disaster	Low	Low	Low	High	Low
	Medium	Low	Medium	High	Low
	High	Medium	High	Medium	Medium
Scenario 2: Terrorist attack	High	Medium	High	Medium	Medium
Scenario 3: Global pandemic	Low	Low	High	Low	High

donors become ill and unable to donate, long-term stocks might be depleted across the country, as seen with the Zika crisis. As such, the extent to which the local shortages can be compensated by importing blood from unaffected areas depends on how widespread the pandemic is and whether areas that have traditionally been net exporters of blood (e.g., the Midwest) are affected by the outbreak. Currently, the Zika virus has not spread to all of areas of the country, which has allowed for redistribution of blood across the system. Therefore, the overall risk during pandemic situations is relatively high.

Availability of Collection Supplies and Reagents

Blood centers are increasingly relying on a few large vendors for their collection and laboratory needs (e.g., blood bags, fractionation supplies, testing reagents).[38] Additionally, a single vendor produces certain blood supplies at very low profit margins.[39] Just-in-time inventory management is increasingly being used to keep supplies lean and costs low.[40] Such an arrangement benefits blood centers by reducing warehousing costs associated with the storage of supplies and helping consumption levels stay in line with stock, which minimizes or eliminates obsolete stock. However, a further reduction in the number of key suppliers could result in increases in market prices if the market becomes uncompetitive. This could be particularly challenging in the market for blood collection suppliers, as many have large barriers to entry, with significant start-up costs stemming from FDA regulations and approvals. Thus, even with a more-consolidated

---

[38] RAND interviews with blood centers and vendors, February 1 through June 30, 2016.

[39] RAND interviews with blood centers and vendors, February 1 through June 30, 2016.

[40] RAND interviews with blood centers and vendors, February 1 through June 30, 2016.

market for blood centers, it would be difficult for blood centers to coalesce to put pressure on suppliers to reduce prices if there were only one or two suppliers for a particular good.

Suppliers or Vendors During Natural Disasters

Although we did not find much empirical evidence pertaining to blood center vendors during natural disasters, relying on a few vendors and just-in-time delivery represents a potential weakness in the supply chain because of the lack of redundancy. Should one vendor become incapacitated or overwhelmed in a disaster, the supply chain could see significant delays or shortages in essential supplies across the country.

Suppliers or Vendors During Terrorist Attacks and Pandemics

Significant delays or shortages in inputs for blood centers become particularly important during a pandemic scenario. Unlike natural disasters or terrorist attacks, in which the threat to essential services comes mainly from physical damage to key infrastructure, the primary risk to services in a pandemic is reduced blood supply from fewer donations and a reduction in workforce in the form of high rates of absenteeism over extended periods of time. As such, shortages in essential staff at vendors to blood centers might cause delays in production of essential supply. Therefore, supply vendors could represent a critical vulnerability to the blood supply chain.

Suppliers or Vendors Risk Assessment

Table 7.4 summarizes the risk that supply vendors pose to the blood system. For natural disasters and terrorist attacks, the risk is ultimately dependent on the location of the disaster—should the disaster incapacitate any one of the vendors, the entire blood

Table 7.4
Risk Assessment of Supply Vendors

	Magnitude of Impact	Supply Vendor Vulnerability	National System Absorption Capacity	Overall Risk Score for Blood System
Scenario 1: Natural disaster	Low	Low	Low	Low
	Medium	Potentially high, depending on location	Low	High
	High	Potentially high, depending on location	Low	High
Scenario 2: Terrorist attack	High	Potentially high, depending on location	Low	High
Scenario 3: Global pandemic	Low	High	Low	High

system would see shortages in essential supplies. During a pandemic, the threat to essential staff who work for the vendors is high. There is little or no redundancy in vendors, so the overall risk posed to the blood system is consequently high.

Availability of Skilled Technicians, Critical Equipment, and Lab Space

The backbone of any industry is the availability and capabilities of a skilled workforce. Skilled nurses, lab personnel, and technicians perform critical and often labor-intensive tasks, such as conducting screening questionnaires, collecting blood from donors, operating apheresis machines, processing and analyzing the collected specimens, testing for diseases, discarding unusable samples, and inventorying.[41] During the past 20 years, there has been a continued decline in the number of skilled workers choosing medical technology and medical science careers. In a recent study, 43 percent of clinical laboratories in the United States reported difficulties in finding qualified job candidates.[42] In the blood banking industry, the vacancy rate in phlebotomy labs is reported at 15.1 percent, 11 percent in blood bank lab personnel, and 11 percent in microbiology testing labs.[43] As such, blood centers might not be able to meet demand during times of surge because of the lack of personnel available or willing to work overtime to meet surges in demand. Additionally, should key individuals become incapacitated from injury or illness during a mass casualty scenario or pandemic, routine blood center activities might be delayed or cease to function effectively. Therefore, the blood center workforce represents a potential weakness in the blood supply chain.

In addition to personnel, blood centers use highly specialized equipment and wet-lab spaces, and these spaces are often subject to strict regulation and inspection. Such equipment is highly sensitive to disruptions in critical infrastructure, such as water and electricity.

Blood System Staffing During Natural Disasters

While we could not find much direct evidence of blood center activities in terms of personnel and equipment following a natural disaster, we believe that the following evidence from terrorist attacks might also be representative of natural disasters.

Blood System Staffing During Terrorist Attacks

Blood centers must have enough trained personnel to screen donors and test donations. As trained personnel are already strained during normal times, most blood centers do not have the capability to handle surges without extensive overtime hours, which can

---

[41] American Society for Clinical Pathology, *The Medical Laboratory Personnel Shortage*, policy statement, April 2004.

[42] HRSA, *The Clinical Laboratory Workforce: The Changing Picture of Supply, Demand, Education and Practice*, Washington, D.C.: HHS, July 2005.

[43] Edna Garcia, Asma M. Ali, Ryan M. Soles, and D. Grace Lewis "The American Society for Clinical Pathology's 2014 Vacancy Survey of Medical Laboratories in the United States," *American Journal of Clinical Pathology*, Vol. 144, No. 3, September 1, 2015, pp. 432–443.

lead to exhaustion, fatigue, and related failure. After the Oklahoma City bombing, the local blood center estimated that 7,000 donors emerged in the first 72 hours, leading to massive lines and delays. The head of the blood center was noted as saying, "People lined up outside the building and waited for hours. Part of handling the disaster for us was finding a way to accommodate all of these donors; we were not equipped to handle that many people. Our staff worked day and night for several days."[44] Similar phenomena were observed after the September 11 attacks,[45] and the nightclub shooting in Orlando.[46]

Additionally, donor surges can lead to an overcollection of blood, leading to future wastages. Because blood is a perishable good, too much blood in the system leads to outdating and waste. It is well documented that U.S. blood centers collected nearly 500,000 excess units of blood after the September 11 attacks, an estimated 250,000 of which were discard.[47] Therefore, blood centers must be willing to turn people away or encourage them to donate at a later date. Although this surge in extra units during times of emergencies may seem to suggest that the blood system is well prepared for public health emergencies, the system faces challenges in efficiently absorbing and managing extra units. More effort to facilitate the handling of extra units so as to avoid wastage is needed.

Finally, donor surges during disasters tend to bring in an influx of first-time donors, necessitating more-rigorous testing for infectious diseases. A surge in volunteers may be accompanied by a higher incidence of donors with transfusion-transmissible infections. After the September 11 attacks, the influx of first-time donors was accompanied by a tripling in the number of blood units infected with potentially serious microbes, including HIV, HBV, and HCV.[48]

Blood System Staffing During Pandemics

Blood center personnel are not immune from a pandemic and may be at a greater risk of acquiring an infectious disease because of their high exposure to a range of people on a daily basis. They may also be concerned about disease contraction from exposure. For example, during the SARS outbreak, only 48.4 percent of health care workers across 47 facilities in a New York metropolitan region said that they would be willing to report to work.[49] Thus, we assumed that there would also be a 30-percent to 50-percent reduction in essential staff at blood centers. Because specialty lab personnel needed to collect, process, and test blood products are already in low supply, such a hit

---

[44] Gilcher, 2001.

[45] Kidder, 2010.

[46] "Blood Donation Lines Grow in Orlando After Shooting," *ABC 7 News*, June 12, 2016.

[47] Schmidt, 2002; GAO, 2002.

[48] Douglas Starr, "Bad Blood: The 9/11 Blood-Donation Disaster," *The New Republic*, 2002, pp. 13–16.

[49] Khan, 2014.

to personnel would have potentially devastating consequences. Effects could include a backlog of blood needing to be tested, processed, or blood-typed.

Blood System Staffing Risk Assessment

Table 7.5 summarizes the risk that essential personnel and equipment pose to the overall blood system. For natural disasters and terrorist attacks, the vulnerability to local personnel or equipment is a function of the overall effect of the disaster. The national vulnerability is low, as the disaster is unlikely to incapacitate equipment and personnel located elsewhere in the country. However, there is a documented national shortage in essential lab personnel, and while people can potentially be relocated in times of need for smaller-scale disasters, the national system has a medium-to-low capacity to absorb local shocks. Therefore, for medium- to high-impact disasters, the overall risk posed by personnel to the blood system is medium to high.

For a pandemic, the national vulnerability of personnel is high. Furthermore, because people across the country are equally likely to get sick, there is little ability for the system to absorb personnel shortages. Therefore, the overall risk score is high.

Status of Critical Infrastructure

From a disaster planning perspective, the status of electricity, IT infrastructure, water, and waste removal are fundamental to the basic activities of a blood center. For example, lack of power or water could result in a shutdown of processing and testing activities. Lack of power could compromise on-site storage facilities, which require refrigeration. Additionally, lack of power could also compromise IT infrastructure, disrupting inventory management. Blood centers, suppliers to blood centers, or hospitals using a single IT infrastructure could also be at a significant risk in the event of computer failures or cybersecurity attacks.

Table 7.5
Risk Assessment of Essential Personnel and Equipment

	Impact	Local Personnel or Equipment Vulnerability	National Personnel or Equipment Vulnerability	National System Absorption Capacity	Overall Risk Score for Blood System
Scenario 1: Natural disaster	Low	Low	Low	Medium	Low
	Medium	Medium	Low	Medium	Medium
	High	High	Low	Low	High
Scenario 2: Terrorist attack	High	High	Low	Low	High
Scenario 3: Global pandemic	Low	High	High	Low	High

Critical Infrastructure During Natural Disasters, Terrorist Attacks, and Pandemics

Natural disasters and terrorist attacks often result in extensive damage to critical infrastructure, potentially incapacitating local blood centers. During pandemic conditions, the overall reduction in workforce in all sectors might lead to delays in routine maintenance and repair work in the electrical and telecommunications grids and water and sewage systems.

Critical Infrastructure Risk Assessment

Table 7.6 summarizes the risk posed to the overall blood system by critical infrastructure. During natural disasters and terrorist attacks, the vulnerability of the local infrastructure is a function of the impact of the disaster. However, the vulnerability of national infrastructure is low, and the system has a relatively high capacity to compensate for local disasters. Therefore, the overall risk is relatively low. During pandemics, the overall risk to infrastructure is not incapacitation but, rather, maintenance during labor shortages. Therefore, the vulnerability is moderate, but the absorption capacity is low, leading to a moderate risk overall.

Storage and Transportation

Depending on the various levels of demand and the geographic location of a hospital, blood centers will make regular shipments of whole blood and components on a twice daily, daily, biweekly, or weekly basis to the hospitals served. In a metropolitan area, most regular shipments are on a daily basis. For outlying rural areas, the shipments may only be weekly. In this process of inventory and distribution management, a blood center must decide (1) its own optimal maintenance inventory levels, (2) its inventory allocation policy, in the event of demands from the hospital blood banks that it serves, (3) its transshipment policy to other blood centers or out-of-network hospitals in the

Table 7.6
Risk Assessment of Critical Infrastructure

	Magnitude of Impact	Local Critical Infrastructure Vulnerability	National Critical Infrastructure Vulnerability	National System Absorption Capacity	Overall Risk Score for Blood System
Scenario 1: Natural disaster	Low	Low	Low	High	Low
	Medium	Medium	Low	High	Low
	High	High	Low	Medium	Medium
Scenario 2: Terrorist attack	High	High	Low	Medium	Medium
Scenario 3: Global pandemic	Low	Medium	Medium	Low	Medium

event of shortages elsewhere, and (4) its recycle policy for moving unused but unexpired blood from one hospital to another.

Blood centers mainly rely on transportation contracts with air and ground delivery services.[50] While not a major consideration during normal times, transportation infrastructure, such as fuel, energy, road conditions, and personnel, are of major importance during disasters. As the vice president of the New York City blood center stated after the September 11 attacks: "All the blood that you could ever need exists somewhere in the country. The trick is making sure that it is in the right place at the right time."[51] Therefore, the crux of the supply chain during disaster times is the ability of units of blood to be transported from one region of the country to a disaster-stricken area.

The transportation and logistics sector is under increasing pressure from an explosion in online sales and a global shift to just-in-time inventories. Pressures on the transportation sector include (1) loss of a skilled workforce; (2) deterioration of existing fleets across the freight, shipping, and transportation sectors; and (3) the overall deterioration of the highway and rail infrastructure. Disasters are likely to exacerbate such problems. As such, transportation demands represent a critical failure point in the blood supply chain. Figure 7.5 demonstrates key influences and decision drivers for the transportation industry.

Figure 7.5
Key Influences and Decision Drivers for the Transportation Industry

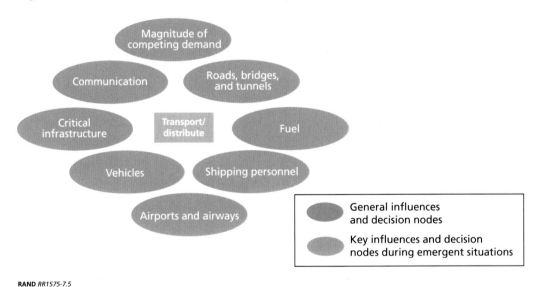

RAND RR1575-7.5

---

[50] RAND interviews with blood centers, February 1 through June 30, 2016.

[51] Kidder, 2010.

Transportation and Storage Concerns During Natural Disasters

Many emergent events, such as storms and blizzards, occur regularly and tend to have minimal effects on transportation systems, such as delays, partial closures, or diversions. Other events, such as earthquakes, hurricanes, and terrorist attacks, can have huge effects on transportation infrastructure. Virtually every sector in our global economy is heavily reliant on the transportation sector. Basic needs, such as the distribution of food, coal distribution to provide electricity, fuel distribution for transportation, and medical supplies, require a working transportation sector. Therefore, there are many competing demands on the transportation supply chain, which could result in delays and shortages in a natural disaster. This could be compounded, depending on the scale of the disaster and the number of entry points into a disaster zone. For example, Hurricane Sandy incited the preemptive shutdown of all airports, ports, and public transit systems in the region. After the storm, it took several days for the system to return to normal operating conditions because of massive flooding, which had substantial effects on relief efforts.[52] Similarly, the 2011 Japan earthquake and associated tsunami led to massive damages in transportation infrastructure, delaying humanitarian aid despite the biggest national repair directive in Japanese history.[53]

Air transportation is often the only feasible mode of transportation for first responders and urgently needed relief supplies.[54] Following an earthquake, tsunami, or hurricane, most roads, rails, and ports become unusable, as they are blocked for days by debris. On the other hand, airports operate in large, open spaces, where debris from a natural disaster can be removed quickly. Furthermore, a runway usually suffers remarkably little damage even from a strong earthquake, such as those experienced in Nepal or Haiti. And even if there are cracks and holes in a runway, modern relief aircraft can typically operate safely in these conditions.[55]

Additionally, local transportation personnel could be injured or incapacitated. As such, drivers might need to be brought in from other locations or recruited from volunteer populations to ship blood products from various blood centers to their point of demand.

Fuel availability also affects the ability of blood to be shipped from outside of a disaster-stricken region. Additionally, competing humanitarian demands often exacerbate fuel shortages. For example, there were massive fuel shortages in the aftermath of Hurricane Sandy that delayed humanitarian aid. Because of its harbor and terminal infrastructure, the oil-and-gas supply chain in the United States is particularly prone to storm surges during hurricanes. At the same time, the supply chain is greatly depen-

---

[52] Todd Litman, "Lessons from Katrina and Rita: What Major Disasters Can Teach Transportation Planners," *Journal of Transportation Engineering*, Vol. 132, No. 1, 2006, pp. 11–18.

[53] Khan, 2014.

[54] Schultz, Koenig, and Noji, 1996.

[55] "Nepal Quake: Airport Customs Holding up Aid Relief—UN," BBC, May 3, 2015.

dent on a secure power supply. During Hurricane Sandy, such infrastructures as pipelines, oil terminals, storage tanks, and filling stations could hardly function because of power outages. Only a small number of installations remained operational with access to backup power systems. As such, there were massive fuel shortages in the aftermath of the storm.[56]

Similarly, when Hurricane Rita hit Louisiana and Texas in 2005, officials ordered the evacuations of coastal cities and provided free bus transportation for nondrivers. Most residents responded to evacuation instructions, which resulted in massive fuel shortages. Exacerbating the problem, many fuel stations ran out of gasoline because fuel truck drivers did not report to work. Some evacuees spent hours searching for fuel. Vehicles failed along the way due to overheating and running out of fuel, further exacerbating evacuation challenges.[57]

For natural disasters, in the post-disaster chaos, law enforcement personnel are deployed to enforce public health orders, secure perimeters of disaster zones, prevent civilian harm, and secure national stockpiles of essential medical supplies. However, such efforts often hamper humanitarian aid. For example, in the aftermath of Hurricane Katrina, the National Guard and local authorities controlled access to New Orleans—civilian humanitarian organizations were barred from the city, hampering relief efforts. Therefore, water, food, equipment, and skilled rescuers were turned back, misdirected, or misused.[58]

Transportation or Storage Concerns During Terrorist Attacks

Issues with local transportation personnel, transportation systems, and deploying public health and law enforcement personnel are similar to those in natural disaster events, but they would depend on the extent to which the terrorist attacks affected transportation infrastructure. While fuel availability is a critical concern during a natural disaster, it is a much lesser concern during local terrorist attacks (unless fuel is the target of such an attack) and pandemics.

Transportation or Storage Concerns During Pandemics

In a pandemic, we can assume a 30-percent reduction in transportation personnel nationwide. Because the transportation workforce is already strained, it may represent a critical vulnerability during this scenario.

The vulnerability of transportation infrastructure is dependent on the ability of the labor force to routinely maintain infrastructure in pandemic situations. Hence, the infrastructure only represents a low vulnerability in this scenario.

---

[56] Laura Nahmias, "Poor Communication Fueled Post-Sandy Gas Shortage," *Wall Street Journal*, March 20, 2013.

[57] Litman, 2006.

[58] Elizabeth T. Boris and C. Eugene Steuerle, eds., "After Katrina: Public Expectation and Charities' Response," The Urban Institute, May 2006.

During pandemic conditions, country, state, and local borders might limit free movement, particularly when directed by public health quarantine orders, to curtail the spread of disease. This could potentially affect the availability of supplies and reagents necessary for blood center operations, as it is estimated that 80 percent of raw materials for lab reagents come from manufacturers located abroad.[59]

During a global pandemic, it is very likely that locally available food, energy, and medical resources will be quickly exhausted, and replacements are likely to be delayed. Because transportation is already strained, a significant reduction in transportation personnel is likely to cripple the distribution of goods across the country from such competing demands that cannot be triaged away.

Transportation Risk Assessment

Table 7.7 summarizes the risk posed by the transportation sector to the U.S. blood system. It is important to note that the capacity of the national blood system to absorb local shocks is irrelevant here because importing blood from unaffected regions to meet surges in demand or local shortages hinges on a working transportation sector. On the other hand, competing demands on the transportation sector become a factor in assessing the overall risk.

Table 7.7
Risk Assessment of Transportation Sector

	Magnitude of Impact	Personnel Vulnerability	Infra-structure Vulnerability	Fuel Vulnera-bility	Competing Demands	National System Absorption Capacity	Overall Risk Score for Blood System
Scenario 1: Natural disaster	Low	Low	Low	Low	Low	N/A	Low
	Medium	Medium	Medium	Medium	Medium	N/A	Medium
	High	High	High	High	High	N/A	High
Scenario 2: Terrorist attack	High	Medium	Medium	Low	Medium	N/A	Medium
Scenario 3: Global pandemic	Low	Medium	Low	Low	High	N/A	Medium

---

[59] Deborah Autor, "Securing the Pharmaceutical Supply Chain," hearing before the Committee on Health, Education, Labor and Pensions, U.S. Senate, Washington, D.C.: Food and Drug Administration, September 14, 2011.

As such, for natural disasters, the overall vulnerability for the transportation sector is a function of the effects from the natural disaster—a large hurricane like Hurricane Sandy can have massive and lasting consequences on transportation. Competing demands are also a function of the severity of the disaster, and therefore the overall risk is consequently dependent on the effects of the disaster.

During terrorist attacks, the transportation sector is less vulnerable overall, unless it is the direct target of the attack. However, there are fewer competing demands during terrorist attacks (i.e., food), and therefore the overall risk is medium.

Pandemics mostly affect personnel, and therefore the overall vulnerability of the transportation sector is low. However, competing demands are potentially very high during pandemics, resulting in a moderate overall risk score.

Hospital Activities and Considerations

Similar to blood centers, the goal of a hospital's blood bank is to maintain availability of blood products while minimizing outdating and costs. In addition, hospitals are responsible for the final blood group–testing, cross-matching, ordering, and transfusing of blood. Figure 7.6 demonstrates the key influences and decision nodes for hospitals and other providers. Many of the same threats that blood centers face in the event of emergencies from infrastructure, transportation, and personnel affect hospitals similarly. In this section, we briefly highlight additional vulnerabilities that hospitals face and discuss evidence from natural disasters, terrorist attacks, and pandemics collectively.

Inventory Management

The short shelf life of blood products necessitates a close linkage between stock inventory and immediate planned use. The size of local inventory is determined by routine day-to-day use, with built-in latitude in anticipation of emergency need. In general, hospitals do not build inventory in anticipation of major events that would require a surge in supply. Rather, hospitals rely on blood centers that maintain excess capacity in preparation for gaining market share and therefore can deliver blood on short notice.

Trained Personnel

Highly skilled technicians are needed for hospital blood banking activities that include cross-matching, inventory management, supplier interface, patient evaluation, and product preparation. As mentioned previously, roughly 15 percent of phlebotomy laboratory personnel positions are unfilled in the United States.[60] As such, trained hospital technicians and other personnel represent a potential weakness in the U.S. blood system during emergent situations.

---

[60] Garcia et al., 2015.

Figure 7.6
Key Influences and Decision Nodes for Hospitals

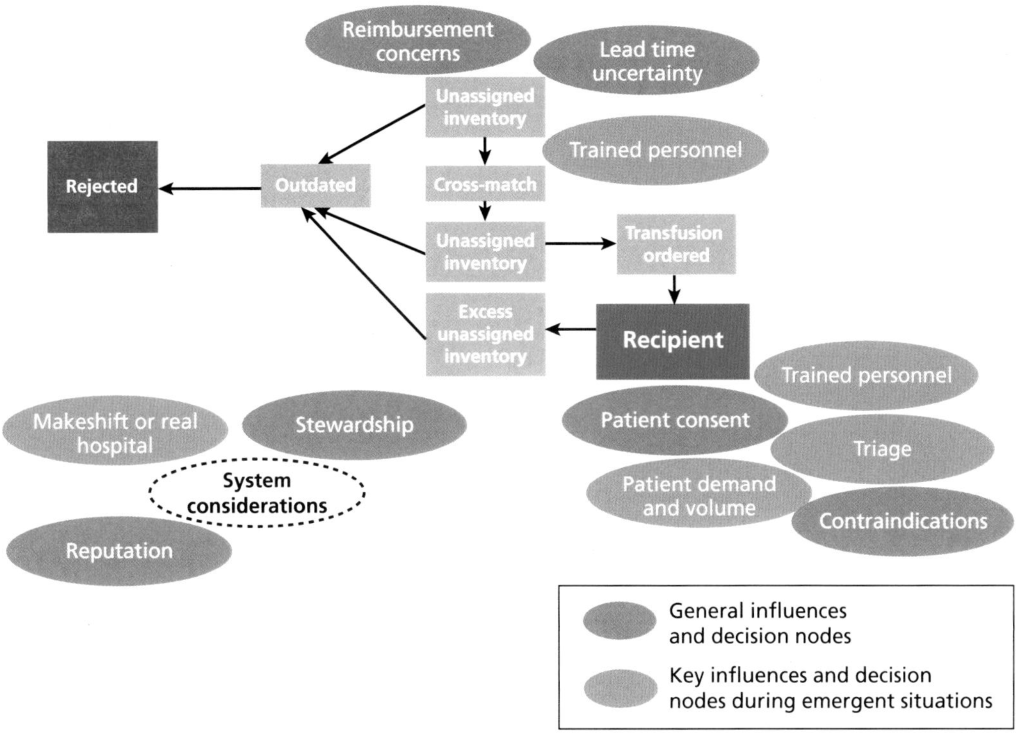

RAND *RR1575-7.6*

Cross-Matching

Cross-matching is the process by which the donor blood type is matched to the recipient blood type. Once a quantity of blood has been ordered and type-matched, it is categorized as "assigned inventory" within a hospital's blood bank. While blood requested for cross-matching by a physician is expected to be transfused, physicians often order more units than necessary to prevent shortages during emergency situations in the operating room or during childbirth. Therefore, when only a certain proportion of assigned blood is transfused, the unused units of blood are returned to free inventory within the hospital.[61]

During times of high demand or such emergent conditions as mass trauma events that necessitate immediate surgical intervention, there may be insufficient time to fully test and cross-match blood samples. In extreme emergencies, when there is no time to obtain and test a sample, group "O" Rh-negative packed red cells can be released.[62] In

---

[61] Williamson and Devine, 2013.

[62] Williamson and Devine, 2013.

such a situation, the clinician must sign a release authorizing and accepting responsibility for the use of incompletely tested products as a lifesaving measure.[63]

Hospital-Level Challenges During Natural Disasters

Although we did not find direct evidence in the United States for demand considerations during natural disasters, evidence from the Japanese earthquake and tsunami suggest that any uptick in demand because of mass trauma is easily balanced by reduction in elective procedures. It was noted that in the immediate aftermath of the disaster, 37 percent fewer transfusions were performed than in predisaster times, and shortages in blood supply were not observed, despite the incapacitation of major regional blood centers.[64]

Hospital-Level Challenges During Terrorist Attacks

Contrary to popular belief, terrorist-related disasters generally do not create immediate blood shortages. U.S. hospitals and first responders have not yet experienced a critical shortage of blood and blood products in the immediate aftermath of a mass casualty incident.[65] This discrepancy can be attributed to a finely tuned national distribution system that enables regional surplus to be transported into areas of greatest need. Medical facilities generally keep a three-day supply on hand as a matter of course, to be used primarily during scheduled surgeries.[66] However, noncritical procedures are usually canceled in the event of a disaster so that all available blood can be directed toward victims.

There have only been a few notable events in the United States that have used more than 100 units of blood in the first 24 to 30 hours following a disaster incident:[67] (1) the collapse of a hotel in Kansas City, Missouri, in 1981; (2) the crash landing of an airplane in Sioux City, Iowa, in 1989; (3) the bombing of a federal building in Oklahoma City in 1995; (4) the 1999 shooting at Columbine High School in Denver, Colorado; (5) the September 11, 2001, attacks on the World Trade Center in 2001; (6)

---

[63]   Juan C. Duchesne, John P. Hunt, Georgia Wahl, Alan B Marr, Yi-Zarn Wang, Sharon E Weintraub, Mary Jo Wright, and Norman E. McSwain Jr., "Review of Current Blood Transfusions Strategies in a Mature Level I Trauma Center: Were We Wrong for the Last 60 Years?" *Journal of Trauma and Acute Care Surgery*, Vol. 65, No. 2, 2008, pp. 272–278.

[64]   Kenneth E. Nollet, Hitoshi Ohto, Hiroyasu Yasuda, and Arifumi Hasegawa, "The Great East Japan Earthquake of March 11, 2011, from the Vantage Point of Blood Banking and Transfusion Medicine," *Transfusion Medicine Reviews*, Vol. 27, No. 1, 2013, pp. 29–35.

[65]   Steven N. Vaslef, Nancy W. Knudsen, Patrick J. Neligan, and Mark W. Sebastian, "Massive Transfusion Exceeding 50 Units of Blood Products in Trauma Patients," *Journal of Trauma and Acute Care Surgery*, Vol. 53, No. 2, 2002, pp. 291–296.

[66]   AABB, *Disaster Operations Handbook*, Bethesda, Md., October 2008.

[67]   Vaslef et al., 2002.

the Sandy Hook shooting in Newtown, Connecticut, in 2012; and (7) the Orlando nightclub shooting in 2016.[68]

These disasters occurred in cities of various sizes at different times of the week and involved different types of injuries. In each case, however, all blood collections were managed locally, and blood from outside sources was not needed. It is worth pointing out that although the blood system has historically been capable of responding to these emergency needs, it is unclear whether this will hold as the industry continues to contract.

Hospital-Level Challenges During Pandemics

While the supply side of the blood supply chain is increasingly strained under pandemic conditions, limiting transfusions to critical procedures and postponing or canceling those deemed elective can significantly reduce demand. However, estimates of demand in such a situation vary. For example, unpublished survey data from clinicians and other experts in the United Kingdom (UK) and Australia suggest that only 10 percent to 40 percent of transfusions are critical, time-sensitive, and "lifesaving."[69] Additionally, recent experiences with blood shortages have demonstrated the reduction in use of blood and blood products without detrimental effects for patients. For example, during the SARS outbreak in Toronto, Canada, RBC use decreased by 25 percent with no harm to patients.[70]

Conclusions

Table 7.8 summarizes the risk scores for key players and decision nodes in the U.S. blood supply chain.

Overall, despite tight forecasting and inventory control, the U.S. blood system has been relatively resilient to disaster scenarios.

We identified several areas of vulnerability in the supply chain, but we note that the following two areas spanned multiple nodes in the system: (1) a shortage of essential personnel and (2) a lack of redundancy in supply vendors. To mitigate the latter, blood centers should consider warehousing essential supplies rather than relying on just-in-time inventory. Additionally, blood centers can advocate for national stockpiles of critical supplies funded by government contracts similar to medical countermeasure contracts. However, mitigation of personnel shortages is more challenging, as such shortages represent a disinclination of people to enter medical science fields. Expansion of educational opportunities, such as apprenticeship programs and electronic learning

---

[68] Brinkmann, 2016.

[69] AABB, 2009.

[70] AABB, 2009.

Table 7.8
Summary of Risk Scores

	Scenario 1: Natural Disaster			Scenario 2: Terrorist Attack	Scenario 3: Global Pandemic
Impact	Low	Medium	High	High	Low
Donors	Low	Low	Medium	Low	High
Blood center reserve stocks	Low	Low	Medium	Medium	High
Vendors to blood centers	Low	High	High	High	High
Blood center personnel and equipment	Low	Low	Medium	Medium	High
Critical Infrastructure	Low	Low	Medium	Medium	Medium
Transportation	Low	Medium	High	Medium	Medium
Demand	Low	Low	Medium	Medium	Low

curricula, may be necessary to boost the workforce. Interventions and employer policies that encourage first responders and medical or laboratory personnel to deploy in the event of emergencies may also be considered.

Second, terrorist attacks and natural disasters are problems of surges in demand coupled with potential local shortages. However, because such scenarios are highly local events, surges in demand caused by trauma-related injuries have historically been absorbed easily by the national system as a whole despite local shortages. Therefore, the crux for such scenarios becomes critical infrastructure and transportation issues, which directly affect the system's ability to move blood both locally and nationally.

During pandemics, supply is the main concern. Shortages in donors and essential personnel at blood centers, vendors, and hospitals can lead to increasing supply shortages over time. However, shortages in supply can be compensated by reduction in nonessential procedures, mitigating potential detrimental impacts. It is important to note that we assessed the impact of a pandemic situation in the absence of other factors that may cause surges in demand. For example, if there were a mass shooting at a time of pandemic crisis, critical shortages in supply might not be able to meet surges in demand.

Finally, in consideration of the insurance value of blood, as discussed in Chapter Six, it is worth highlighting that there is little evidence on what an appropriate level of surge capacity in the system should be. We have noted industry norms for blood centers and hospitals to maintain an inventory that would suffice to match the blood supply for a given blood center or hospital for a period of three days,[71] but a more-thorough and more-precise analysis estimating local and national emergency needs could inform emergency preparedness efforts and discussions about excess capacity in the system that serves as a public health good. In such an analysis, a critical evaluation of the system's most significant vulnerabilities would help to determine how to also address those vulnerabilities. For example, the ability to redistribute blood around the system locally or nationally appears to be a substantial challenge in several emergency scenarios. Efforts to quantify how much stockpiled blood would be needed to alleviate that risk could inform both emergency planning and government interventions to support such stockpiling. Cost considerations would also be necessary; in particular, maintaining a surge capacity would largely be a fixed cost and, as the market continues to contract, the average fixed cost for maintaining this surge capacity would actually increase. In sum, a thorough analysis and definition of the appropriate quantity of blood necessary to maintain a surge capacity and a cost-benefit analysis are needed to ascertain what policy efforts might be considered to mitigate risks described in this chapter.

---

[71] Magali J. Fontaine, Y. T. Chung, F. Erhun, and L.T. Goodnough, "Age of Blood as a Limitation for Transfusion: Potential Impact on Blood Inventory and Availability," *Transfusion*, Vol. 50, No. 10, 2010, pp. 2233–2239; Michelle L. Erickson et al. "Management of Blood Shortages in a Tertiary Care Academic Medical Center: The Yale–New Haven Hospital Frozen Blood Reserve," *Transfusion*, Vol. 48, No. 10, 2008, pp. 2252–2263.

CHAPTER EIGHT

Potential Innovation in Business Models

Introduction

Demand for blood products has declined, and although the blood industry has closed facilities, there still appears to be excess capacity in the system. This, at least partly, explains recent declines in the prices for blood products. Existing blood collection entities operate using a variety of business models and are adapting in different ways as they struggle to find ways to remain financially sustainable. The predominant business model approaches that will remain or emerge as the blood market reaches a new equilibrium will have significant effects on many aspects of the nation's blood supply. This chapter focuses on the potential effects of using alternative business models to supply the nation's blood and examines the implications that such changes would have on the sustainability of the blood system.

This chapter begins with a brief review of the current market structure. We then describe three different business models that might play significant roles in the near future. To get a sense of which future scenarios are more likely, we consider what forces are likely to promote or discourage these various business models. Finally, we consider how the expansion of each alternative model would affect prices, quality, sustainability, and the resilience of the nation's blood supply. This includes the ability of those systems to respond to shocks and fund R&D.

Current Market Structure and Business Models

Both hospitals and blood centers face varying degrees of direct and indirect costs involving inventory management, shelf life, staffing, and wastage. Costs vary by region, and they have been increasing as new pathogens emerge and as the FDA adds testing and safety requirements. Meanwhile, demand has been slowly declining over time, a trend that is likely to continue as more hospitals begin to use patient blood management systems.

Who Are the Big Players?

There are 131 unique organizations in the United States that operate as blood collection facilities. Much of the U.S. blood supply is collected by a few large organizations. ARC collects and processes about 40 percent of the U.S. blood supply and has at least one affiliated blood establishment in about 78 percent of all health care markets (or HRRs) in the United States.[1] Blood Systems Inc. (BSI) covers another 10 percent of the market. ARC has the scale to include pathogen testing under its organizational umbrella. High fixed costs make it inefficient for smaller blood centers to test their own blood, so they typically subcontract these services to a larger testing organization, such as ARC or Creative Testing Solutions. Some larger centers have expanded and consolidated testing services beyond their previous scale to achieve new efficiencies. Smaller blood centers often coordinate supply purchases and the exchange of blood products through member organizations, but each blood center remains an independent organization. The largest blood center membership organization is BCA, whose 45 members collect 30 percent of the U.S. blood supply. One reason that independent blood centers might work together is to help control costs. For example, HemeXcel is a GPO that reduces supply costs for its members, including BSI. Together, they collect about 25 percent of the nation's blood supply. Many of those same members also jointly own Creative Testing Solutions, which provides blood-testing services.

Our analysis of FDA Form 2830 data merged with health care market-level data (see Chapter Three for more details) suggests that, on average, there are about five blood collection or blood bank facilities in any given health care market in the United States (see Table 8.1).

Predominant Business Models

A variety of business models are used to meet hospitals' demands for various blood products and services, ranging from large full-service national centers to patchworks of smaller regional and local centers and organizations that collaborate to provide the blood products desired by hospitals. With demand from hospitals generally exceeded by the available supply of blood products, competition drives prices down in most areas, although pockets of low competition remain. Falling prices cause lower or negative margins that might soon drive some blood centers out of business. Some blood centers are trying to wait out what is seen as a rough market that will eventually subside, while others are changing their business models in response to these market changes. As a start to discussing the sustainability and reliability of a market based on alternative business models, this section highlights three business models that might expand in the near future.

---

[1] Authors' calculations using FDA Form 2830 data. See Chapter Three for more details.

Table 8.1
Mean Number of Blood Establishment Entities in U.S. Health Care Markets, per Hospital Referral Region

	Mean	Standard Deviation
Collection	2.57	2.96
Hospital blood banks	1.77	2.79
Nonhospital blood banks	0.59	0.78
Warehouse	0.19	0.87
Processing	1.91	2.19
Distribution	0.43	0.69
Testing	0.09	0.35
Other	0.29	0.70

NOTES: Based on 306 HRRs; see Chapter Three.

Nationally Integrated Organizations

National integration involves geographically dispersed blood centers collaborating under a common organizational structure. A nationally integrated organization could be formed through internal expansion, acquisitions, mergers, or partnerships between organizations. The national integration model best represents the relationships between blood centers and hospitals in the current blood system, with varying degrees of intensity in collaboration. At one end of the spectrum are large single organizations, such as ARC, which sometimes expand their own networks or acquire other blood centers to increase their geographic presence and market share. On the other end are affiliations between networks of independent blood centers, such as BCA, HemeXcel, Versiti, and National Blood Collaborative, which have grown by bringing more members into their networks. The distinction is not sharp; for example, BSI might bring additional organizations into its network of subsidiary or affiliated blood centers via acquisitions or via its membership in the HemeXcel organization, while at the same time those organizations might be expanding through mergers or acquisitions. Currently, the national blood market includes several nationally integrated organizations, and the existence of one nationally integrated organization does not necessarily preclude the existence of other nationally integrated organizations.

Merging blood centers under a single organization, whether formally, as with ARC blood centers, or informally, as with other blood center cooperatives, saves money by consolidating excess capacity, increasing bargaining power when procuring supplies, and enabling organizations to exploit geographic variation in collection costs, including the cost of donor recruitment. In other words, a blood center that operates in markets with both relatively high and low costs of blood production could produce more blood in the low-cost market to be exported to the high-cost market. That blood center also be in a better position to offer lower prices to hospitals in the high-cost market by subsidizing the high-cost market with proceeds from the low-cost market. Some blood centers (e.g., ARC) may already do this. Merging also increases member centers' ability to sell to large hospital networks that often prefer to contract with a single blood supplier. Merging geographically dispersed blood centers under a single organizational structure does not necessarily imply that only one organization is the sole source of blood products in their respective regions.

Some have suggested that the blood supply industry may be best served by a single national blood system, akin to a natural monopoly (see discussion in Chapter Six). There are examples of single national systems from other nations. Typically, in such markets, government intervention is necessary to prevent market failure; this could be done either through a public-run system or through a heavily regulated private system. The distinction would be important, as public versus private national systems might have different appetites for risk and a different focus on urban versus rural regions and would face different incentives for innovation. Either way, it is unclear whether there would be public or political support in the United States for such a completely publicly run system. The process of arriving at a single national organization from the present market structure would also require significant time to resolve organizational complexities. Merging might require assimilating computer systems, closing some collection locations, and potentially renegotiating various contracts. However, further national integration in the U.S. blood sector might still allow a competitive market environment, as organizations could expand without becoming the only source of blood products. As connecting geographically distant markets and transporting blood products between them becomes easier and more widely practiced, it becomes increasingly difficult for one organization to monopolize a region.

Most large blood centers and blood center organizations are engaging in national integration, so further expansion of this business model is a realistic possibility.

Independent Local Organizations

The provision of blood products by independent local or regional organizations is an alternative to the nationally integrated business model. Each geographic area (or perhaps health care market) would have an independent blood center that acts as the sole provider of blood products to local hospitals. At the most extreme level of localization, there are some examples of hospitals collecting their own blood and some examples of hospitals closely coordinating with a local blood center partner organization. Movement of blood products between local or regional blood centers could still occur to address shortages. However, such exchanges would be more limited than between blood centers under a single organization because of limited information about the geographic availability and pricing of blood products, as well as the additional costs of arranging transactions between separate organizations. In the localized organizations model, testing and processing blood would likely remain subcontracted to larger or specialized organizations because testing processes involve large investments in equipment that are most cost-effective for processing large quantities of blood.

Because localized organizations cannot as easily achieve economies of scale or exploit geographic price differences, they are often at risk of being underpriced by alternative models. Yet some hospitals worry that contracting with a nationally integrated organization may reduce competition, with the resulting monopoly causing even higher future prices. Some hospitals also value the responsiveness and dependability of their local blood centers, which is why they invest in those close relationships. While this model often has higher per-unit blood purchase costs, a hospital is more likely to have some influence over the business practices of the blood center that serves it and is also more likely to engage in a dialogue with blood center experts who can make suggestions to improve logistics or transfusion safety.

Brokerage

An alternative to national integration or localization models is a brokerage model, in which a third party helps to connect buyers and sellers of blood. The broker never explicitly owns the blood, but it is instead a network for connecting sellers and buyers, and is typically financed by a fee on each completed transaction. Examples of brokerage models include the NBE and Bloodbuy. This is similar to, but distinct from, a middleman business model in which the business buys blood from the blood center and resells it to hospitals or another blood center, with the middleman bearing the associated risk and gaining the associated profits.

Hospitals often desire to continue working with the same blood center for purposes of consistency, reliability, flexibility, or trust. If the blood center from which a hospital orders is short on a particular blood product, that blood center might order the particular blood product from another blood center and then sell that product forward to the hospital. In other cases, hospitals might turn to sources beyond their primary long-term contract partner when that blood center is short on a particular product or hospitals need additional blood beyond amounts agreed to in the long-term contract. The extent to which brokerage models support transactions between two blood centers versus between a blood center and a hospital varies significantly. One brokerage organization reported that 60 percent of its transactions were between two blood centers and 40 percent were between a blood center and a hospital, while another reported that 20 percent of its transactions were between two blood centers and 80 percent were between a blood center and a hospital. The prevalence of brokerage transactions between two blood centers relative to brokerage transactions between a blood center and a hospital might be subject to further change as the percentage of nationally integrated or localized organizations evolves. Nationally integrated firms internally arrange this geographic shifting of blood products, which would lower the demand for brokerage services. An increase in the share of the blood market held by local organizations would probably increase the demand for brokerage services to balance out local supply shortages.

Although the majority of transactions supported by the brokerage model are for stat orders, a brokerage can also help connect hospitals and blood centers to form longer-term contracts. Hospitals can also use the brokerage model to place standing orders for particular blood products at particular frequencies and pricing conditions. Placing repeat orders through a brokerage model could, in theory, completely displace long-term contracts between a single hospital and a single blood center. Such a model has the attractive qualities of capturing savings from geographic cost differences and providing price transparency that can lead to more-competitive pricing for both blood centers and hospitals. However, such benefits can come at the expense of other benefits associated with face-to-face interactions and known local suppliers. The desire for repeated business means that brokerage firms have strong incentives to ensure that the quality of the blood products sold in their transactions meets the expectations of the market participants.

Once parties interact through the brokerage model setting, they could barter outside of the brokerage platform. Legal disputes have arisen in middleman models over whether transactions directly between a buyer and seller would have occurred without the third-party connection. In theory, the same issues could arise in brokerage models, which is one reason that brokerage models may prefer that the buyer and seller remain unknown to each other until after the transaction is agreed upon. Brokerage firms also argue that double-blind transactions help to lower prices by encouraging competition and help to optimize connections between hospitals and blood centers by prohibiting the habit of working only with previously known organizations.

Which Factors Promote Various Models?

It is not clear which of these business models is likely to dominate the U.S. blood market in the near future. To date, the nationally integrated organizations appear to have gained share compared with local independent organizations, and a relatively new national brokerage platform (Bloodbuy) appears well positioned to expand. This section examines the factors that could contribute to shifting the market in the direction of a particular model (Table 8.2).

Hospital Mergers

The trend of hospital mergers is sometimes cited as one factor that will drive blood centers toward their own horizontal mergers, as many larger hospital networks or systems prefer to source their blood from a single, large supplier. Some blood centers have argued that hospital consolidation has contributed significantly to downward pressures on the market price for blood. In our descriptive analysis of health care market

Table 8.2
Which Factors Will Benefit or Challenge Various Business Models?

	Nationally Integrated Organization	Local Independent Organization	Brokerage
Further hospital mergers	Comparative advantage	Comparative disadvantage	Unclear
Decrease (increase) in transportation costs	Comparative advantage (disadvantage)	Comparative disadvantage (advantage)	Comparative advantage (disadvantage)
Increased safety concerns	Variable	Comparative advantage	Comparative disadvantage
Increased use of electronic inventories	Comparative advantage	Comparative disadvantage	Unclear
Mobile collection of specialty blood products	Variable	Variable	Variable

data linked to the FDA registry of blood establishment entities, we found significant positive correlations between the number of unique blood establishment facilities and (1) the number of hospitals in the market, 0.62 ($p = 0.00$) and (2) the number of inpatient discharges, 0.82 ($p = 0.00$). However, the correlation between the number of unique blood establishments and the level of hospital concentration in the market, measured as the hospital HHI,[2] is negative, -0.48 ($p = 0.00$). When we adjusted for other market-level characteristics,[3] we found a similar negative association, as shown in Figure 8.4.[4] This negative association is not necessarily indicative of a causal relationship, but it is suggestive that as the hospital market becomes less competitive, there seem to be fewer blood establishments. However, the level of hospital concentration in any given market might also affect blood establishments' decision to participate in the market. Thus, it could be the case that blood establishments are sorting into markets with a more-competitive hospital market. It is also important to keep in mind that the number of blood establishments, although likely correlated with the volume of blood

---

[2] HHI is calculated as the sum of the market shares squared for each hospital in the HRR and ranges from 0 to 1, in which the larger value represents a more highly concentrated market. For example, an HRR with ten hospitals with equal shares of the market (HHI = $10 \times (0.1)^2 = 0.1$) is less concentrated (more competitive) than a market with two hospitals with equal shares of the market (HHI = $(0.5)^2 + (0.5)^2 = 0.5$). We define share of the market as equal to the number of Medicare inpatient discharges at each hospital divided by the total number of Medicare inpatient discharges in the HRR.

[3] We adjusted for the following market-level measures: the number of Medicare enrollees, population, the number of acute care hospital beds per 1,000 residents, the number of hospital-based registered nurses, the number of FTE hospital employees per 1,000 residents, the number of surgical discharges per 1,000 Medicare enrollees, and the total number of inpatient discharges.

[4] For the full set of results, see the appendix.

Figure 8.1
Predicted Number of Unique Blood Establishments, by Level of Hospital Market Concentration

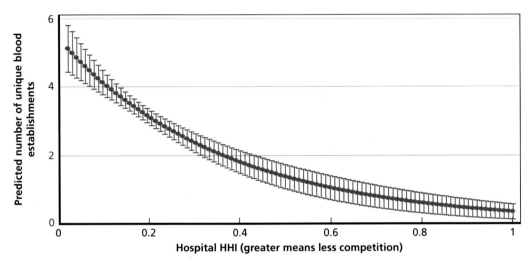

SOURCE: FDA data merged with Dartmouth HRR data.
NOTES: Points represent estimated number of unique blood establishments in a market for a given level of hospital competition (HHI). Bars represent 95-percent confidence intervals.
RAND RR1575-8.4

collected, does not necessarily reflect the total stock and flow of blood in a particular HRR.

Aside from the association of hospital consolidation with price, large hospital systems often prefer to work with blood centers that are large enough to service all hospitals in the system, creating an incentive for centers to merge. Larger hospital systems could increase administrative efficiency by working with the same blood center for most or all of their hospitals. However, most hospital systems are still regional, so all the hospitals in their system could be served by blood centers that are already regional. Thus, at present, administrative efficiency gains from horizontal mergers are most likely from having one organization serve multiple regions rather than from matching the hospital's scale. If more hospital systems merge to span broader geographic areas, this could increase pressure on blood centers to match hospitals' geographic breadth.

Hospital mergers might make it simpler and more administratively efficient for the hospital to work with suppliers of similar scale. In particular, if increased hospital mergers are paired with increased use of electronic inventories, the hospital-specific requests could be automated or at least brought under a single system. Together, these trends could significantly reduce administrative costs for large, nationally integrated blood centers. Both increased hospital mergers and the increased use of electronic inventories seem quite plausible in the immediate future. Nationally integrated firms would be better aligned to benefit from these potential cost savings than local organizations and some brokerage models. However, the extent to which servicing a single hospital system reduces costs for the blood provider, relative to the costs of servicing several separate systems, is limited. Even if administrative costs are reduced for the blood center, these costs are a small portion of the costs of supplying blood products to meet each hospital's unique standing orders and stat delivery requests.

Changes in Transportation Costs

At about 10 percent of the total costs associated with producing a unit of blood, transportation costs are approximately equal in magnitude to the various administrative and IT costs. Changes in transportation costs could also have a large effect in shaping the business models of the future U.S. blood market.

If transportation prices decline, business models that rely on transportation to exploit regional cost differences could potentially flourish at the expense of local and regional blood centers. This would be the case if, for example, blood centers that operated in multiple markets were subsidizing prices in markets with high blood transportation costs from blood collected in markets with lower transportation costs. With reduced transportation costs, the amount of those subsidies would decline. Regional differences in the price of blood would decline, and it would be easier to meet local surges in demand or compensate for local declines in supply.

Although declines in transportation costs would likely increase the extent to which certain low-cost regions of the country were net exporters, the complete disappearance of local blood centers would be unlikely. While modern air transportation means that blood can be shipped across the country in a matter of hours, some organizations report that shipping can be delayed or complicated during holidays. Hospitals can preemptively stock up before delays or preemptively arrange post-holiday deliveries, but this can be trickier for blood products with short shelf lives, such as platelets. Hospitals would still rely, at least to some extent, on a local or regional supply. Occasional limitations in transportation availability mean that no amount of geographic differences in collection costs will result in blood products being exclusively collected in a single region of the country, although both nationally integrated firms and brokerage models will exploit these geographic cost differences as much as possible.

Conversely, increases in transportation costs would tend to favor local organizations. The geographic exchange of blood would decline, and price differences across regions would increase.

Safety Concerns

Safety concerns have previously transformed how blood was supplied in the United States. Although blood centers might want to increase their investments in testing and safety, declining profit margins make it difficult for blood centers to fund any testing beyond what is required by FDA. If concerns over the safety of the U.S. blood supply outpace FDA's ability or inclination to regulate, hospitals could become more willing to pay for additional testing beyond FDA requirements, particularly if they were concerned about liability. The INTERCEPT PRT for platelets or plasma is another, more-recent example, as it is not yet required by FDA. However, many blood centers are interested in investing in PRT if hospitals are willing to pay a high-enough price to compensate for the expense, and a small number of blood centers are already offering it. Hospitals, blood centers, and FDA are all closely monitoring babesia outbreaks in the northeast United States, which might result in hospitals' willingness to pay higher prices for unrequired babesia testing or blood from another region.

Although any of the models discussed earlier could potentially provide increased testing, risk-averse hospitals might favor getting blood from blood centers that they can more closely monitor and trust. Some of the blood centers we interviewed suggested that local independent blood centers charged higher prices than nationally integrated blood centers, but they typically offered hospitals more-direct involvement in testing investments that met the hospital's preferences. However, a brokerage or nationally integrated model does not necessarily preclude blood centers from selling blood products with additional testing or processing beyond what is required by FDA. Hospitals could also still monitor or build trusting relationships with blood centers in other regions.

Technological Innovations

A variety of technological innovations could alter how blood is collected, tracked, matched, and used. The implications vary depending on the innovations. Next, we discuss two potential innovations with direct implications for how blood centers are organized.

Electronic Inventories

A variety of technological innovations could also shape the ability of various business models to be successful. Electronic Inventory Management (EIM) can help hospitals reduce wastage, track their supplies, and reduce administrative labor. And, as discussed earlier, the expansion of electronic inventories could further reduce administrative costs associated with blood provision for all business models. However, high up-front costs and IT complexity might limit the demand for EIM. In 2012, preliminary cost estimates of EIM were as high as $575,000 per year for a managed service contract.[5] Enabling a hospital to share EIM access with blood centers or a brokerage might require one or both sides to upgrade their IT infrastructure.

Nationally integrated organizations would benefit in particular, as electronic inventories allow one administrator to serve more hospitals. Independent local organizations would benefit from the increased efficiencies as well, but the high fixed costs

---

[5]   M. F. Murphy, E. Fraser, D. Miles, S. Noel, J. Staves, B. Cripps, and J. Kay, "How Do We Monitor Hospital Transfusion Practice Using an End-to-End Electronic Transfusion Management System?" *Transfusion*, Vol. 52, No. 12, 2012, pp. 2502–2512.

might discourage investment relative to nationally integrated organizations that can benefit from the same system across a larger number of hospitals.

For brokerages, the effect of electronic inventory tracking is unclear. Successful inventory management might reduce stat orders through more-efficient monitoring of stock and personalized need forecasts and reduce the revenue of brokerages. On the other hand, electronic inventories could be used to automatically post orders to brokerage markets and, in doing so, might make it significantly easier and cheaper for hospitals to use a brokerage. Automated ordering could reduce the cost of spot orders, making brokerage spot markets an alternative to long-term contracts as a primary source of blood products for hospitals. Some brokerages already offer the ability for hospitals to set up recurring orders, and automating the process could be done easily. The effect depends partly on hospital preferences, but overall it should increase efficiency. If hospital managers are averse to automated or electronic ordering of blood, electronic inventory monitoring would smooth working with nationally integrated firms and long-term contracts more than brokerages and spot markets.

Mobile Collection

Operating a brick-and-mortar collection facility is costly for blood centers and requires busy donors to come to the blood center. Mobile blood collection is often cheaper than at brick-and-mortar facilities, but collecting specialty blood products, such as plasma, requires complex equipment that is more-easily housed in fixed centers. Innovations that make mobile collection easier, particularly for specialty blood products, could reduce the gap in collection costs between blood centers with highly concentrated pools of donors and blood centers with more dispersed pools of donors. Which business model such innovation would favor depends on the extent to which a center's donor base is dispersed.

Impacts of Expansions of Alternative or Nascent Business Models

In this section, we examine the possible effects of the expansion of these business models on prices, quality, and the sustainability of the U.S. blood supply (Table 8.3).

Impact on Prices

Cost is a critical concern for hospitals, blood centers, and suppliers involved in the U.S. blood market. Although the market price (that hospitals pay to blood centers) has shifted downward over time, it is unclear where the new equilibrium price will be as the market evolves.

Expansion of nationally integrated organizations might allow blood centers to leverage geographic cost differences and gain economies of scale through a single organizational structure. If this results in reduced competition among blood centers through mergers or closures of blood centers in a given market, prices could increase.

Table 8.3
How Would the Expansion of Each Model Impact Particular Characteristics of the U.S. Blood System?

Blood System Characteristic	Nationally Integrated Organization	Local Independent Organization	Brokerage
Prices	Decrease given competition Increase without competition	Increase	Decrease
R&D investment	Moderate	Moderate or minimal	None
Ability to provide specialty products or testing	High	Varies	High
Responsiveness to hospital needs	Moderate	High	Varies
Spread or isolate risk?	Spread	Isolate	Spread

However, the magnitude of such an increase depends on what happens to the demand for blood (e.g., if it continues to fall, prices might increase but by less).

If there is an increase in independent local blood centers, then the market concentration or competition among blood centers would increase, which could drive prices down further. However, in markets dominated by one or two independent local blood centers, prices might increase, as those entities are less able to exploit geographic variation in blood production costs or enjoy economies of scale. Thus, although the organizational structures have implications for costs at the blood center level, the overall market structure will play an important role in determining what happens to the market price for blood.

As noted previously, the brokerage model potentially allows blood centers to sell across geographic markets more efficiently, which may yield higher prices in some markets. However, the brokerage model also facilitates better price transparency, which presumably will yield more competitive pricing.

Impact on R&D

One benefit of the expansion of large, nationally integrated firms is that they are better positioned to increase spending on various types of R&D that make blood supplies safer, cheaper, and more reliable. Investment in R&D can be expensive, and the benefit per unit of blood produced can be small. Large, nationally integrated firms have enough financial capacity to invest in this type of R&D. The level of competition in a given blood center market, however, may influence blood centers' decisions about R&D investment. In noncompetitive markets, blood centers might have little incentive to invest in R&D, as they do not need to differentiate themselves from competitors.

There might be investment in R&D that produces cost savings, but there is little incentive to pass on savings to customers. On the other hand, large, nationally integrated firms can also more easily raise prices in noncompetitive markets to fund such investments. In more-competitive markets, blood centers' profit margins will be lower, which might discourage R&D investment, but innovation in the market might also allow blood centers to differentiate themselves and charge higher prices. In general, there could be concern about innovation becoming publicly available, introducing the classic "free rider" problem, whereby blood centers or entities that did not invest in the R&D enjoy the benefits as technological innovation diffuses. To the extent that innovation is a public good, the government can fund this type of R&D to avoid this problem.

Smaller, independent local organizations may have fewer resources to pursue R&D investments independently. As the number of organizations performing R&D increases, it can also become more difficult to avoid redundancies of effort—a topic that we further explore in the following chapter on international best practices. The most likely form of financing research under an expansion of vertically integrated blood centers would be national organizations, public or private, that pool funds from independent blood centers or elsewhere to address national research priorities.

Impact on Ability to Provide Specialty Products or Testing

Another important concern of both hospitals and blood centers is the ability to obtain or provide specialty blood products. Not only do some patients require unique blood products, but this demand might need to be filled on short notice.

Nationally integrated organizations and brokerage organizations might have an advantage in providing specialty blood products or facilitating their exchange. Both are able to draw on a diverse set of donors and collection facilities in different regions. Both systems are well designed and incentivized to identify the nearest available specialty product and the fastest method of providing it, as well as forecasting where such demands might arise.

Local independent organizations are less likely to have a full suite of specialty products available within their organizations. Local independent organizations are likely to invest in producing specialty products if the hospitals they work with frequently need those products; otherwise, such investments are not cost-efficient. Local independent blood centers have long relied on coordination with other blood centers to fill demand for specialty blood products. These coordination mechanisms are likely to take the shape of secondary market brokerage models. Unlike the expansion of nationally integrated organizations, an increased market share of local independent organizations does not necessarily run counter to the brokerage model. In that scenario, the question becomes the extent to which brokerage models will serve the secondary market versus the primary market.

Hospitals might also desire specific testing processes. Demand for testing beyond FDA regulation tends to be limited to centers directly affected by the adverse effects of not using that technology. Because testing has large returns to scale, testing is likely to remain centralized in any of these models, with little differences in organizational ability to meet unique pathogen testing needs (beyond differences in R&D investment). Blood centers often cite a desire to use advanced pathogen testing and treatment methods, but they suggest that there is low hospital demand for this. It might be the case, however, that blood centers are not as effective as test developers or testing organizations would be at explaining the benefits of additional testing to hospitals. Investments in new testing techniques are declining across the market overall because developers' expected return on investment is uncertain unless and until FDA mandates the test.

Impact on Blood Center Responsiveness and Dependability

Independent local blood centers reported that the value they provide involves more than just delivering a commodity at the lowest cost. They tended to pride themselves on maintaining responsive and dependable relationships with the hospitals they serve. Hospitals and blood centers in this model are more likely to engage in joint activities beyond the delivery of blood. Blood centers can support hospital fellowships and training for hospital staff, and hospital staff can serve on the blood center's board of directors. Business and scientific consulting services can flow in either or both directions. Independent local blood centers often have more full-time staff in the local region, enabling them to spend more time engaging with their hospital partners.

The role and importance of these services are more complicated in nationally integrated and brokerage models. Some large hospital systems prefer the benefits of matching with a single large provider. Nationally integrated firms argue that despite hospital systems buying in bulk for lower prices, the economies of scale are not as large as hospitals expect because the nationally integrated blood center still works with each hospital independently to meet its unique needs. However, smaller independent local blood centers displaced by expanding horizontally integrated blood centers often lament a "race to the bottom" where price per unit is minimized at the expense of other benefits.

The importance of these blood center services varies across brokerage models. Some models are extremely concerned about personal relationships. Trust and networking are viewed as absolutely critical for knowing whom to call to connect supply and demand. Alternatively, brokerage models can be much more focused on efficiency. Brokerage software can be focused on connecting supply and demand while quickly and efficiently sorting blood products by price, type, testing, source, and other such quantifiable factors. Valuing service quality can sometimes be viewed as impeding the efficient functioning of markets. Hospitals and blood centers are seen as overvaluing the trust they place in their current suppliers, stuck in the habit of working with one party, while different blood centers are willing to provide the same services at a lower price or a different hospital is willing to purchase those services at a higher price.

Impact on Risk

Effects of particular concern in this report are the sustainability of various market structures and their ability to respond to shocks and other sources of risk.

Both nationally integrated organizations and brokerage models reduce the risk associated with external local or regional shocks on the supply of or demand for blood. A shortage in one region is resolved by shifting extra supply from other regions. Modern transportation of blood products makes this process rapid enough to resolve most localized shocks. Independent local blood centers are more exposed to local shocks. A regional weather event or other natural disaster might delay collection, leaving vertically integrated firms unable to collect blood for several days. Such situations as this make some form of geographically diffuse secondary markets critical for reducing the risk of blood shortages. Similarly, independent local blood centers will have more difficulty handling excess supply without the risk of wastage. On the other hand, independent local blood centers are less exposed to shocks outside of their region. Disruptions to the transportation network, particularly the air transportation network, could significantly hamper nationally integrated organizations and brokerage models that rely more heavily on rapid national transportation.

Another source of risk is the organizational capability of the U.S. blood market as a whole to collect the amounts of blood needed nationally at any point in time. Some interviewed organizations felt that declining demand left the market as a whole with too much capacity to collect and process blood, and the closure of some blood centers was seen as a painful but inevitable part of market correction. At the same time, other interviewed organizations saw the continued existence of this "excess" capacity as critical for insuring a reliable supply of blood at all times. The expansion of nationally integrated organizations or the movement of brokerage models into the primary market would likely result in additional closures of blood centers. At present, the risk of national shortages because of the closure of blood centers appears minimal. However, it is not clear whether the closures of blood centers would continue until new stable levels are reached or whether closures would continue until shortages become more frequent, forcing another transformation of the market.

Conclusions

What is the outlook in the immediate future for the business models used to meet the nation's blood demand? In general, due to their own incentives, most hospitals have focused on finding cost savings. Cost-sensitive hospitals and declining demand for blood have put pressure on all business models, but particularly on the independent local blood centers. Additional closures and mergers should be expected, with an immediate future of very lean profit margins for all blood centers. Eventually, further closures would start to reduce capacity to collect and process blood relative to demand, forcing prices back up. Across the different business models, some organizations are thinking strategically about how their behavior now will affect their status after the excess supply issue has been resolved, and they are likely to continue expanding in the future. Other organizations have been largely reactionary, with little interest in proactively altering the market or with limited ability to engage in proactive planning beyond waiting for prices to rise. These organizations are less likely to expand or be prepared for the future market. Although many individual organizations will grow or shrink in market share, without further changes, no single organization or business model is likely to dominate the entire market in the immediate future. Demand for brokerage services is increasing as hospitals seek out low-cost sources for blood products and as independent local blood centers seek ways to collaborate to survive on thinning profit margins. All business models could benefit from creatively thinking about how to navigate real or perceived trade-offs between price efficiency and service benefits.

What does this outlook mean for sustainability in the immediate future? ARC has suggested that an additional $1.2 billion in excess infrastructure still exists in the market,[6] but the length of time it will take for enough blood centers to close to reduce excess capacity is unclear. Proactive funding for research from the market is unlikely during this period, creating challenges and requiring government intervention for both the present Zika crisis and future blood safety issues until the market stabilizes—an issue that we explore more fully in the following chapters. There is some worry that long-term damage will be inflicted on the market because declines in demand for certain job skills during this supply correction could create a shortage of skilled workers when the market stabilizes. This could impede technological and safety advances even after demand, prices, and margins stabilize or begin to rise. While safety records suggest that large safety failures or supply shortages are unlikely, FDA needs to remain vigilant and aware that, for the immediate future, its regulations are the driving force for the uptake of existing pathogen testing technology, which, in turn, determines incentives for investment in researching future pathogen testing technology. On the other hand, however, a reorganization of the market that reduces redundancy, although potentially painful in the short term for some entities, could result in a more-stable and more-efficient market in the long term. Workforce shortages could become less problematic with fewer centers serving a particular market, for example.

How these changes in the business models used to supply the nation's blood will affect hospitals and ultimately influence patient welfare depend on many factors. Policy efforts to maintain a well-functioning market, both nationally and locally, will be important for keeping prices competitive in the long term. The extent to which hospitals will change their procedure prices in response to changes in the price of blood is unclear. Insured patients do not presently bear these costs directly and are likely to be relatively insensitive to price changes for lifesaving blood, so the financial effects

---

[6]   Hrouda, 2015.

on patients are likely to be small and indirect at most. It is possible that the closure of blood centers would increase the risk of supply shortages, although there seems to be adequate slack built into the system.

In summary, how the structure of the market will evolve is unclear, and the effects of changes at both the blood center level and more broadly across the market can have systemwide implications. Consolidation in a particular market yielding a regional (or even national) blood center monopoly could drive up prices, depending on what happens with the demand for blood. There are also concerns that, without government intervention, the current trajectory for the U.S. blood system is a painful reorganization that will continue to drive costs down, and all surviving blood centers will be in poor financial shape. Although evidence does suggest that there is too much redundancy in the system, there are potential solutions that could reduce excess capacity without devastating the system and without excessive government intervention. Market-induced consolidation or reorganization also does not necessarily imply a noncompetitive market. Thus, we should consider aspects of the market that are not well functioning as areas where the government can step in to facilitate changes that will ensure a sustainable and safe blood supply in the long term. We discuss possibilities in Chapter Ten.

CHAPTER NINE

Best Practices from Other Nations' Blood Systems

Introduction

Although the U.S. blood system is unique in many respects, in part because of the broader U.S. health and legal environment, there are lessons to be learned from other nations' blood systems that U.S. policymakers could potentially apply here. In this chapter, we examine best practices from foreign countries to generate ideas that could help improve the U.S. blood system by increasing safety, lowering costs, reducing shortages or waste, or increasing cost-effective research and innovations. Policy changes that achieve these goals are likely to increase the overall sustainability of the U.S. blood system.

When comparing several other nations' blood systems, we do not attempt to make general statements comparing one entire system to another: This chapter will not analyze the broad advantages and disadvantages of entire blood systems. Instead, we focus on specific practices, which we loosely refer to as "elements" of blood systems. This approach highlights best practices that have the potential to incrementally improve the U.S. system. The specific system elements that we decided to highlight include practices related to HV, regulations governing blood-related medical devices, and government support for R&D. Based on the practices we have observed in other countries, we recommend that U.S. policymakers and managers of U.S. blood system organizations work together to:

1. Build a more effective national HV program by
   a. increasing participation in the U.S. HV reporting system
   b. ensuring adherence to HV case definitions to improve data accuracy
   c. centralizing HV data aggregation, analysis, and results dissemination.
2. Improve the regulatory environment for medical devices by
   a. increasing the speed and decreasing the cost of regulatory approvals for medical devices to the extent possible without reducing safety
   b. harmonizing with or converging to internationally prevalent blood safety standards.

3. Coordinate and encourage investments in R&D by
    a. sustaining or expanding government blood-related R&D investments
    b. more closely coordinating the investments of blood centers, suppliers, and government funders.

Methods

The focus of this chapter is on describing individual practices in other blood systems rather than entire blood systems. There are significant challenges involved in replicating blood systems in the United States from other countries, including different models of health care system organization and financing; different structures and responsibilities for public health entities; different resources along the vein-to-vein donation, processing, and transfusion process; and different cultural and social norms.

In this chapter, we focus on blood system practices that appear to have produced positive results in at least one foreign country. The term *best practice* is, by definition, a practice that has demonstrated positive results. We then assess whether the best practice is (1) applicable to the U.S. blood system and (2) feasible in terms of implementation in the United States.

Research questions: The following research questions guided our research design.

1. How do specific policies or practices observed in foreign blood systems differ from U.S. practices, and which of these differences appears to have produced positive results? In other words, what best practices can we observe in foreign blood systems?
2. Are any of these best practices applicable to the U.S. system, and would it be feasible to implement them here?

Criteria for applicability to the U.S. blood sector: We consider a best practice to be applicable to the U.S. blood system when at least some aspect of the practice is currently not widely adopted in the U.S. system and when that practice could potentially improve the sustainability of the U.S. system.

Criteria for feasibility of implementation in the U.S. blood sector: When we determine that a foreign best practice could be applicable to the blood sector, we then assess the feasibility of implementing the practice in the U.S. blood system. We consider a best practice's implementation in the United States to be feasible primarily if it represents an incremental change in policy or law, rather than an overhaul of the existing U.S. system or laws. If the foreign best practice is applicable to the U.S. blood sector and its implementation is also feasible, then we present and discuss the best practice here.

Criteria for country selection: We focused on a subset of economically advanced nations most comparable to the United States in terms of funding for the blood system and market size. We used national health spending per capita as a proxy for blood system funding; we used total population as a proxy for blood market size. This narrowed our list to ten countries with populations of more than 24 million people and 2014 per capita health expenditures above $2,500[1] at purchasing power parity. We then narrowed this list of large, developed nations to those with abundant English-language research describing their blood systems. Finally, we identified three general types of blood systems—state-run, quasinational (Red Cross), and mixed—and included two of each type, on the assumption that maximizing the diversity of system types would increase the probability of finding unique best practices. Our final list includes six nations from four continents: two with state-run blood systems (the UK and Canada), two that rely exclusively on the Red Cross (Australia[2] and Japan) for blood collection, and two with varying degrees of reliance on privately run blood banks (Germany and Italy).

First, we describe how these six blood systems compare with the United States in terms of size, structure, and evolution. We then present best practices observed in these nations' blood systems that appear applicable to and implementable in the U.S. system.

Limitations of our methodology: Although we applied systematic criteria for selecting comparison countries and for determining whether a best practice—once identified—should be included in this chapter, we did not employ systematic methods for identifying all potentially relevant practices, nor for ranking the practices that we did identify. We relied primarily on interviews with blood sector experts from blood centers, suppliers, and the U.S. government to identify foreign best practices that might be worth researching, and we were able to determine through further research whether several of these possible best practices were applicable to the U.S. system and whether their implementation in the United States might be feasible. We believe that this produced a practically useful list of foreign best practices, but we cannot be certain that we have identified all potentially relevant best practices that this sample of foreign nations may be capable of providing. Nor did we prioritize the list of potential best practices.

When describing a foreign best practice, we depended on examples from some nations within our sample more than others. Although each of our six comparison nations is mentioned at least once in the following discussions, they are not afforded equal coverage. This is partly because of the uneven availability of literature on each nation's blood system and partly a result of random chance. This opens up the possibility that our researchers ended up weighing the experiences of some comparison nations more heavily than others. For example, it is likely that we have researched more

---

[1] World Bank, "World Bank Open Data," undated.

[2] Australia is in some respects a "state-run" blood system that delegates some operations to the Red Cross.

thoroughly and cited the Australian blood system more than we have the Italian blood system.

Brief Overview of Foreign Blood Systems

Next, we examine specific research questions related to the six nations we have selected, and we describe how the six nations compare with the United States in their past evolution and current function (Table 9.1).

Surveying the general structure of these nations' blood systems, we observe that all of them are much smaller than the U.S. system and that large foreign organizations, such as the JRCS, are roughly comparable in size to the largest U.S. blood collection organization (ARC). Some smaller foreign organizations, such as CBS or ARCBS, are comparable in size to the second- or third-largest blood organizations in the United States (such as BSI).

Germany and Italy are structurally most similar to the United States, in that they rely on many blood organizations (or collections of affiliated blood centers, such as the Red Cross) to collect and process blood. After World War II, Germany, Italy,

Table 9.1
General Structure of Seven Nations' Blood Collection Systems

Country or Region	Blood Collection Organization(s)	System Structure
Australia	National Blood Authority (NBA) licenses to Australian Red Cross Blood Service (ARCBS)	State-run and Red Cross
Canada (except Quebec)	Canadian Blood Services (CBS)	State-run
Quebec	Héma-Québec	State-run
Germany	German Red Cross, state agencies (mostly university hospitals), and private commercial blood banks	Red Cross and blood banks
Italy	Italian Red Cross and many blood banks	Red Cross and blood banks
Japan	Japanese Red Cross Society (JRCS)	Red Cross
UK—England	National Health Service Blood and Transplant (NHSBT)	State-run
Wales	Wales Blood Service (WBS)	State-run
Northern Ireland	Northern Ireland Blood Transfusion Service	State-run
Scotland	Scottish National Blood Transfusion Service	State-run
United States	ARC and many independent blood centers	Blood banks

and Japan all reestablished national Red Cross organizations that worked alongside independent and commercial blood banks to collect and process blood.[3] For example, by 1963, corporations or foundations ran more than half of Japan's blood banks, and JRCS ran 16 of the 55 blood banks. However, by 1974, Japan had abolished all commercial blood banks, partly in reaction to transfusion-related infections and partly to establish a 100-percent–voluntary blood donation system.[4] Japan still allows corporate participation in plasma fractionation via a joint venture between JRCS and Benesis Corporation,[5] but it otherwise maintains a Red Cross monopoly on blood collection and processing. Germany and Italy, in contrast, maintain mixed systems that include both the Red Cross and other blood centers.

Unlike the other blood systems in our sample, Australia, Canada, and the UK nationalized most parts of their blood systems. Canada did so in 1998 when it created the CBS and Héma-Québec[6] in response to a tainted blood scandal that implicated the Canadian Red Cross (CRC) in supplying products carrying HIV and HCV.[7] Under the new system, the CRC ceased collecting blood,[8] Héma-Québec took over blood collection in Quebec, and CBS took over in all other Canadian provinces. All Canadian provinces and territories except Quebec now have health ministers who serve as members of CBS, and they also appoint a board of directors to manage the organization. CBS's business decisions are only somewhat independent from the government, as the government appoints all board members, provides overall funding and overall health priorities, and approves the CBS budget.

Australia relied on local branches of the Red Cross to handle its blood supply beginning in 1929. The various Red Cross state and territory blood services later amalgamated to form ARCBS in 1996.[9] Australian federal, state, and territory governments created NBA[10] in 2003, which pooled national and subnational funding to pay for all blood and centralized all policies related to blood safety and supply management.[11] Unlike in Canada and Japan, we could not identify any particular crisis that moti-

---

[3] ARC, "Significant Dates in Red Cross History," undated-b.

[4] Japanese Red Cross Society, *Blood Services 2015*, Minato-Ku, Tokyo: Blood Service Headquarters, 2015.

[5] Japan Blood Products Organization (BP). Benesis is a subsidiary of Mitsubishi Tanabe Pharma Corp.

[6] Canadian Blood Services, A Report to Canadians 2007/2008: Transforming Canada's Blood System, Ottawa, Canada: The Office of Strategy Management, 2008.

[7] "Canada's Tainted Blood Scandal: A Timeline," CBC News, October 1, 2007.

[8] Canadian Red Cross, "A Time of Change: 1990–1999," undated.

[9] Australian Red Cross Blood Service, "History," undated.

[10] Office of Parliamentary Counsel, *National Blood Authority Act 2003*, July 19, 2016; NBA, *National Blood Authority, Australia, Annual Report 2014–15*, Canberra, October 7, 2015b.

[11] Australian Ministry of Health, National Blood Agreement Between the Commonwealth of Australia and the States and Territories, 2003.

vated Australian policymakers to alter the national blood system, and despite the creation of NBA, Australia continues to contract ARCBS to handle all domestic blood collection.[12] Similar to Japan and Canada, Australia also contracts a private corporation (Commonwealth Serum Laboratories CSL Behring) to manufacture most plasma-derived products, and it imports some products from abroad to meet any shortfalls in supply.

The UK nationalized its blood system much earlier and without the impetus of tainted blood tragedies. The UK established the National Blood Service in 1946, which later merged with UK Transplant in 2005 to become NHSBT.[13] NHSBT serves England and Wales and serves more than 85 percent of the UK population, with smaller regions maintaining separate state-run blood collection organizations in Scotland, Northern Ireland, and Wales.

Market Size and Donor Intensity

Of the 164 countries that provided 2008 data to WHO,[14] the ten largest consumers of blood transfusions (by volume) were the United States, China, India, Japan, Germany, the Russian Federation, Italy, France, the Republic of Korea, and the UK. Four of the six nations we selected rank among these top ten, with Australia and Canada ranking close behind (graphed in Figure 9.1).

Five of the six nations that we studied rank similarly to the United States in per capita blood donations, all having more than 30 whole blood donations per 1,000 population. Only Japan has significantly lower donor intensity, having 20 to 29.9 whole blood donations per 1,000 population.[15]

Best Practices from Other Nations' Blood Systems

We identified three best practices from other nations' blood systems that we found were applicable to the United States and feasible to implement: more effective HV programs, an improved regulatory environment for medical devices, and more coordination in R&D. These best practices relate to elements of each blood system rather than to each system's overall structure, because only system elements—not entire structures—can be feasibly transferred to the United States. Although U.S. successes are not the focus of this chapter, we note that the U.S. blood system already functions very

---

[12] NBA, "Overview: Ensuring Supply," undated.

[13] National Health Service, "History," undated.

[14] WHO, "Blood Safety: Key Global Fact and Figures in 2011," Fact Sheet 279, June 2011a.

[15] WHO, 2011a.

Figure 9.1
Whole Blood, Units Collected in Most Recent Year Available

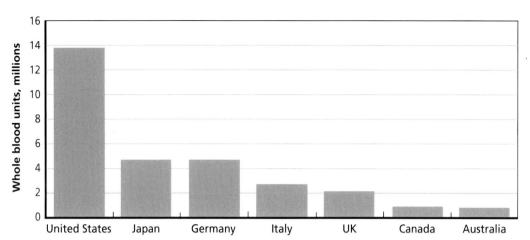

SOURCES: RAND estimates based on available literature, including (Japan) Japanese Red Cross Society, 2015; (Canada) Canadian Blood Services, Centre for Innovation Progres Report 2014-2015, Ottawa, Canada, Centre for Innovation, June 29, 2015 (combined with Hema-Quebec, "Research and Development at Hema-Quebec: An Overview, 2014, p. 34); HHS, 2011b, p. 9; (Italy, Germany, UK, and Australia) European Directorate for Quality of Medicines and Healthcare 2013 report, p. 24.
RAND *RR1575-9.1*

well in most respects, and many best practices observed in other countries are already practiced in the United States. Next, we identify some elements of foreign blood systems that U.S. policymakers and regulators could consider adopting to incrementally improve the sustainability of the U.S. system.

Best Practice 1: Effective Hemovigilance Programs

The emergence of posttransfusion HIV/AIDS, hepatitis, and other adverse health events caused by blood transfusions resulted in several organized, nationwide attempts in the 1990s to measure the frequency of and address such outcomes. These efforts originated in Japan, France, and the UK[16] and are now known as HV. There appears to be general consensus among HV experts that the U.S. HV system is in its infancy and is less effective than are other nations' HV programs.[17]

In this section, we examine what lessons U.S. policymakers and regulators might learn from other nations' HV programs. It is clear from other nations' experiences that

---

[16] Nidhi M. Bhatnagar and Maitry D Gajjar, "Hemovigilance: Need of the Hour," Biennial Journal of GAPM, undated; Hidefumi Kato, Motoaki Uruma, Yoshiki Okuyama, Hiroshi Fujita, Makoto Handa, Yoshiaki Tomiyama, Shigetaka Shimodaira, Yoshiyuki Kurata, and Shigeru Takamoto "Incidence of Transfusion-Related Adverse Reactions per Patient Reflects the Potential Risk of Transfusion Therapy in Japan," *American Journal of Clinical Pathology*, Vol. 140, No. 2, 2013, pp. 219–224.

[17] Roger Y. Dodd and Louis M. Katz, "Qui custodiet ipsos custodes?" *Transfusion*, Vol. 55, No. 4, 2015, pp. 693–695.

effective HV systems can identify transfusion-related problems and measure the effectiveness of interventions designed to address these problems (see Table 9.2). For example, Paul-Ehrlich-Institut (PEI) analysts in Germany were able to measure incidents of immunogenic transfusion-related acute lung injury (TRALI) reactions both before and after September 2009, when new measures were introduced to decrease TRALI reactions. Their data confirmed that these new measures were effective in reducing the number of TRALI reactions.[18] It is also clear from historical experiences in Japan and Canada (see the "Brief Overview of Foreign Blood Systems" section) that before strong HV programs were established, transfusion-related adverse events occurred that hurt confidence in the national blood system, necessitating large structural reorganizations. The application of foreign best practices may improve HV data availability and reliability, thereby increasing researchers' ability to identify and address adverse blood transfusion outcomes occurring in the United States. Any improvement in our ability to identify and reduce transfusion-related adverse events will bolster the sustainability of the U.S. blood system by helping to avoid crises such as those that occurred in Japan and Canada.

Increasing Participation in the HV Reporting System

The lack of external funding, a relatively late start compared with other nations, staff and resource constraints within hospitals, and the voluntary nature of the U.S. system have limited HV system participation in the United States. Work began on the U.S. Biovigilance Network's NHSN HV Module in 2006[19] as a public-private collaboration with HHS, CDC, and organizations involved in blood collection, transfusion, tissue and organ transplantation. The United States had no official national HV system until 2008, when NHSN HV began pilot trial operations,[20] and it was not until 2010 that health care facilities began voluntary enrollment in the HV Module.[21]

---

[18]   Annette Lohmann, Jochen Halbauer, Frau Cornelia Witzenhausen, Frau Klaudia Wesp, Herr Olaf Henseler, and Brigitte Keller-Stanislawski, *Paul Ehrlich Institut (PEI) Federal Institute for Vaccines and Biomedicines, Haemovigilance Report of the Paul Ehrlich Institut 2010,* Assessment of the Reports of Serious Adverse Transfusion Reactions Pursuant to Section 63c, AMG, Arzneimittelgesetz, German Medicinal Products Act, 2010, p.4.

[19]   AABB, undated-b; Centers for Disease Control and Prevention, *The National Healthcare Safety Network (NHSN) Manual: Biovigilance Component Hemovigilance Module Surveillance Protocol, version 2.2,* Atlanta, Ga.: Division of Healthcare Quality Promotion, National Center for Emerging and Zoonotic Infectious Diseases, 2016.

[20]   National Blood Authority Haemovigilance Advisory Committee, Australian Haemovigilance Report, data for 2011–12 and 2012–13, NBA, 2013; Pierre Robillard, "Hemovigilance Systems," Canadian Blood Services PowerPoint presentation, 2008, slide 45.

[21]   Alexis Harvey, Sridhar V. Basavaraju, Koo-Whang Chung, and Matthew J. Kuehnert, "Transfusion-Related Adverse Reactions Reported to the National Healthcare Safety Network Hemovigilance Module, United States, 2010 to 2012," *Transfusion,* Vol. 55, No. 4, 2015, pp. 709–718.

Table 9.2
Overview of HV Programs for Seven Nations

Country, Region or Group	HV Organizations	HV Program Name	Voluntary or Mandatory	National, Regional, or Center-Based
Australia	National Blood Authority (NBA), National Haemovigilance Advisory Committee (HAC)	National Haemovigilance Program	Voluntary[a]	National and regional
Territories (Queensland, Victoria, Tasmania, etc.)	ARCBS Regions, BloodSafe, Blood Watch, Transfusion Safety Program, and others	Voluntary[b]	Regional	
Canada (including Quebec)	Public Health Agency of Canada (PHAC)	Transfusion Transmitted Injuries Surveillance System (TTISS)	Voluntary	National
European Union (EU)	2002 EU Blood Directives	European Hemovigilance Network	Varies (e.g., see Germany, Italy, and UK in following rows)	National
Germany	PEI[c]		Mandatory	Center-based
Italy[f]	National Blood Centre (Centro Nazionale Sangue)	National Haemovigilance System supported by SISTRA (Sistema Informativo dei Servizi Trasfusionali)	Mandatory	National and regional
UK	NHSBT, Medicines and Healthcare Products Regulatory Agency (MHRA)	Serious Hazards of Transfusion (SHOT)	Voluntary	National
Japan	JRCS, Surveillance Committee for Safety of Blood Products in the Blood Advisory Council advises Ministry of Health, Labour, and Welfare (MHLW)	Haemovigilance System of the JRCS	Medical institutions voluntarily report to blood centers, JRCS reports to government are mandatory[d]	National
United States	AABB, HHS's CDC National Health Safety[e]	U.S. Biovigilance Network's NHSN, HV Module	Voluntary[g]	National
ARC	ARC	ARC Hemovigilance Program	Voluntary	Center-based

Table 9.2—Continued

Country, Region or Group	HV Organizations	HV Program Name	Voluntary or Mandatory	National, Regional, or Center-Based
BSI[h]	BSI	Donor Vigilance Program		

[a] Reporting is voluntary, but National Safety and Quality Health Service (NSQHS) Standards mandate that hospitals have systems in place for recognizing and reporting transfusion-related incidents and adverse events; Sunelle Engelbrecht, Erica Wood, and Merole F. Cole-Sinclair, "Clinical Transfusion Practice Update: Haemovigilance, Complications, Patient Blood Management And National Standards," *Medical Journal of Australia*, Vol. 199, No. 6, 2013, pp. 397–401; Erica M. Wood, Lisa J. Stevenson, Simon A. Brown, and Christopher J. Hogan, "The Australian Hemovigilance System," *Hemovigilance*, Wiley-Blackwell, 2012, pp. 209–219.

[b] Engelbrecht et al., 2013.

[c] B. Keller-Stanislawski, A. Lohmann, S. Günay, M. Heiden, and M. B. Funk, "The German Haemovigilance System–Reports of Serious Adverse Transfusion Reactions Between 1997 and 2007," *Transfusion Medicine*, Vol. 19, No. 6, 2009, pp. 340–349.

[d] Hitoshi Okazaki, Naoko Goto, Shun-Ya Momose, Satoru Hino, and Kenji Tadokoro, "The Japanese Hemovigilance System," in R. R. P. de Vries and J.-C. Faber, eds., *Hemovigilance: An Effective Tool for Improving Transfusion Safety*, Wiley-Blackwell, Oxford, UK, 2012, pp. 159–167.

[e] Separately, all U.S. health organizations are required to report to FDA any adverse transfusion events that result in death. Other reporting requirements exist for state health departments and others.

[f] Giuliano Grazzini and Simonetta Pupella, "Setting Up and Implementation of the National Hemovigilance System in Italy," in Rene RP De Vries and Jean-Claude Faber, eds., *Hemovigilance: An Effective Tool for Improving Transfusion Safety*, 2012, pp. 204–208.

[g] FDA does require reporting of fatalities in blood donors and recipients and has proposed a rule to require reporting of serious adverse events

[h] Hany Kamel, Marjorie Bravo, Brian Custer, and Peter Tomasulo, *Donor Vigilance: Five-Year Journey of Continuous Process Improvement*, Blood Systems, 2011.

Total transfused components under surveillance in the HV Module[22] more than doubled from 2010 to 2012, but they rose from only 2.1 percent to 4.5 percent of components transfused nationally during that time. Participation in NHSN is confidential, so CDC is unable to publish a list of enrolled facilities, but it is still clear that the number of enrolled facilities constitutes a small proportion of all eligible health care facilities performing transfusions in the United States.

Many strategies, some derived from the HV experiences of other nations, have been suggested to improve participation rates in the U.S. system. Possible strategies include legally mandating participation, simplifying reporting requirements and otherwise reducing reporting burdens, and attracting participants by making the system more useful to users. Modifications to the U.S. HV Module protocol reporting requirements in January 2013 reportedly reduced the required reporting burden by approximately 50 percent.[23]

---

[22] Harvey et al., 2015.

[23] Harvey et al., 2015.

The experiences of other nations indicate that it is possible to achieve high participation rates without making participation mandatory. The UK's SHOT program, which began in 1996, is one such voluntary system with a voluntary participation rate of 99.5 percent among National Health Service organizations. By 2014, there were only seven nonreporting (low and medium blood use) National Health Service Trusts/Health Boards.[24] The UK demonstrated a steadily increasing number of reports submitted to the SHOT system from 2006 to 2014.

Participation in Canada's TTISS is also voluntary and widespread. TTISS has been monitoring adverse reactions related to the transfusion of blood since 1999;[25] by 2010, the participation rate of hospitals providing transfusion services was 80 percent to 100 percent in 11 provinces and territories, while only one province had a participation rate of less than 50 percent. The volume of transfusions that TTISS monitored can also measure TTISS coverage: From 2006 to 2012, the TTISS network monitored approximately 80 percent of transfusions in Canada. Australian HV participation rates are similarly high, with all provinces and territories except for Western Australia voluntarily reporting regional data to the NBA National Haemovigilance Program.[26]

Japan has a well-established HV system, which officially began in 1993[27] under the auspices of JRCS. Under this mandatory system, hospitals and centers offering transfusion services have established HV systems that share information with the JRCS.[28]

German blood centers, which include the Red Cross and many others, report HV data to PEI,[29] which collected data on approximately 95 percent of all transfused RBC concentrates during 2006 and 2007.[30] This high level of participation has allowed PEI analysts to rapidly identify and minimize risks in the German blood system. Only in Italy is the fragmentation of the blood supply more pronounced than in the United States and Germany, with numerous blood establishments that have only recently begun to consolidate. Italy established an HV system in 2009 that collects data on all

---

[24] Medicines and Healthcare Products Regulatory Agency (MHRA) and Serious Hazards of Transfusion (SHOT), *Annual SHOT Report*, Serious Hazards of Transfusion, 2014.

[25] The pilot program began in 1999 and expanded across most of Canada by 2005, according to Julie Ditomasso, Yang Liu, and Nancy M. Heddle, "The Canadian Transfusion Surveillance System: What Is it and How Can the Data Be Used?" *Transfusion and Apheresis Science*, Vol. 46, No. 3, 2012, pp. 329–335.

[26] NBA, 2013.

[27] Kato et al., 2013.

[28] Kato et al., 2013; Okazaki et al., 2012.

[29] Keller-Stanislawski et al., 2009. Blood components fall under German drug law, so they are covered under pharmacovigilance. However, for transfusion aspects, hemovigilance is applicable.

[30] Keller-Stanislawski et al., 2009.

adverse events for both recipients and blood donors, proving that HV data participation can reach high levels even in an otherwise fragmented blood system.[31]

Ensuring Adherence to HV Case Definitions to Improve Data Accuracy

The U.S. HV system not only suffers from low participation rates, but it also does not sufficiently monitor adherence[32] to the case definitions that organizations use when reporting HV data. As a result, U.S. HV data are likely to be less accurate than some foreign countries' HV data. Because U.S. HV participation is voluntary and data are managed under conditions that ensure confidentiality for reporting organizations, data validation and reporter training are difficult. Each facility owns the data it enters into the HV Module, which are shared with the CDC for public health surveillance purposes as a requirement of participation in NHSN but not shared publicly.[33]

Appropriate case definitions appear to be in place: In 2016, AABB updated its Standards for Classifying Adverse Events to require blood banks and transfusion services to use definitions conforming to international standards.[34] However, when reports are submitted to CDC through NHSN, there is no mechanism at CDC to directly review the submitted data with those providing the reports. A lack of funding exacerbates this challenge—currently no resources external to participating hospitals have been provided for validation of input data.[35]

One effort to monitor U.S. adherence to case definitions occurred in 2014 under the auspices of the Center for Patient Safety (CPS), which is a patient safety organization developed by AABB. Hospitals reporting to NHSN can participate in CPS, which explicitly allows CPS to receive and review data submitted to NHSN. This mechanism has made possible some retrospective review of the validity of reported data by CPS members, and this particular review examined the first three years of data reported to the NHSN HV Module. Of the 14 reports of transfusion-transmitted bacterial infections, the review panel found that five did not meet the case definition. The panel also examined 42 reported pulmonary cases and six "definitive" TRALI reports, but it agreed on only one. Twenty-seven transfusion-associated circulatory overload (TACO) cases were reported, but the panel agreed with only four case definitions and agreed that there were insufficient data to support a report of TACO for 20 of the cases. They concluded that training and education were probably not adequate to improve the current system.

---

[31] Email from Giuseppina Facco, M.D., National Haemovigilance Officer, National Blood Centre, National Institute of Health, Rome, Italy, to authors, August 28, 2016.

[32] Dodd and Katz, 2015.

[33] CDC, NHSN, 2016.

[34] AABB, "Response to Comments Received to the 30th Edition of Standards for Blood Banks and Transfusion Services," undated-c.

[35] Dodd and Katz, 2015.

Self-paced training presentations for HV reporters are currently available on the NHSN Biovigilance Component website, which must be reviewed prior to participating in the HV Module. CDC also provides webinar and in-person training opportunities for current NHSN participants.[36] However, U.S. studies[37] continue to confirm that inconsistent interpretation of case definitions and underreporting of cases and denominators occur, and that simplification of case definitions and improved training for reporters might help. One study that tested 11 U.S. facilities participating in the HV program and 11 that were not participating found that, despite all participants using the same delineated definitions, there was considerable variability in HV responses.[38]

Other nations have made more progress in improving the accuracy and adherence to case definitions in their HV systems. For example, Australia's NBA published new required data elements in August 2015 for the Australian Haemovigilance Minimum Data Set, using definitions taken from national and international standards.[39] The NBA emphasized a crucial step that is largely missing in the United States: data validation. According to the NBA document, "adverse events are investigated, validated and reported at the local level. States and territories are responsible for validating the data before submission to the NBA."[40] This validation process includes the review and validation of the adverse event and might also include the review of severity and "imputability" scores. The reported adverse event might undergo several levels of review (such as initial review and specialist review) until the data issues are resolved.

In Japan, JRCS performs similarly thorough HV validation. JRCS' headquarters assigns 150 medical representatives to blood centers nationwide, and the blood centers report all moderate to severe cases of adverse reactions and infectious disease transmissions. For each of these cases, JRCS headquarters investigates the causal relationship to transfusion.[41] Since 1996, JRCS has even stored 11 years of samples of all blood donations, which enables it to further investigate and verify the causal relationships between blood and adverse reactions or infectious diseases.

Other nations in our sample have made similar progress in improving the quality of their HV data. In Quebec, for example, participation in the HV system includes the involvement of a transfusion safety officer in the investigation of suspected reactions[42]

---

[36] CDC, 2016.

[37] Harvey et al., 2015.

[38] J. P. AuBuchon, M. Fung, B. Whitaker, and J. Malasky, "AABB Validation Study of the CDC's National Healthcare Safety Network Hemovigilance Module Adverse Events Definitions Protocol," *Transfusion*, Vol. 54, No. 8, 2014, pp. 2077–2083.

[39] NBA, "Australian Haemovigilance Minimum Data Set," Canberra, Australia, August 2015a, p.4.

[40] NBA, 2015a, p.5.

[41] H. Okazaki, "The Benefits of the Japanese Haemovigilance System For Better Patient Care," *ISBT Science Series*, Vol. 2, No. 2, 2007, pp. 104–109.

[42] Harvey et al., 2015.

who aids in the validation of data. Unless the United States expands data validation steps, interpretation of data from the U.S. system will continue to prove difficult.[43]

Centralizing HV Data Aggregation, Analysis, and Results Dissemination

Collecting HV data of sufficient quantity and quality is a necessary, but insufficient, step toward identifying and addressing adverse events in a blood system. Someone must also aggregate and analyze these data and disseminate findings, or the system might fail to maintain high levels of quality and usefulness. Although CDC and AABB provide some analysis of HV data, the United States has no government-funded national organization that regularly accesses, analyzes, and disseminates data from all existing U.S. HV programs. The U.S. system remains fragmented[44] in that various subnational and national organizations require separate reporting on transfusion-related deaths and injuries, while such large blood centers as ARC and BSI have developed and maintained their own HV systems, mainly to demonstrate the efficacy of changes in management and safety measures.[45]

HV experts generally argue that aggregating and centrally analyzing HV data carry more advantages than disadvantages. One challenge of centralization is that people with no prior knowledge of transfusion medicine often staff national-level agencies that aggregate and analyze the data, so the transfusion community initially looks on these agencies with distrust. Furthermore, centralized bureaucracies often handle HV as part of a much larger portfolio, so they might not prioritize HV. However, if such an agency consults and hires transfusion experts and begins with a pilot to establish trust and credibility,[46] these challenges can be overcome. On the plus side, public health governance of national HV data and analysis allows the blood system to tap people with extensive knowledge in surveillance methodology, database management, and analysis. It also provides a degree of legal and financial security that might be missing from smaller, fragmented HV networks.[47]

Other nations' experiences prove that the existence of multiple HV data collection organizations need not hinder the pooling and centralized analysis of data. For example, Australian surveillance systems have been established at a jurisdictional (regional) level, and these report to a national HV framework.[48] NBA's HAC receives funding from federal, state, and territory governments and has the capacity to analyze data and generate reports and recommendations. HAC produced its first national HV

---

[43] Dodd and Katz, 2015.

[44] Blood Systems Research Institute, *BSRI Program Review*, BSI, 2011.

[45] Dodd and Katz, 2015.

[46] Robillard, 2008, slides 40 and 42.

[47] Robillard, 2008, slides 40 and 42.

[48] Engelbrecht et al., 2013.

report in 2008,[49] and its most recent 2015 report provides data from all Australian states and territories, except Western Australia. Estimates of infectious and noninfectious hazards are also reported periodically by ARCBS,[50] which receives funding from the national, state, and territorial governments.

Most Canadian hospitals or sites voluntarily report data to a provincial or territorial office, and some report directly to PHAC. Provinces and territories transfer data to PHAC under the TTISS agreement, and it acts as the central repository for all HV data collected in Canada.[51] PHAC reconciles, analyzes, and publishes the data approximately two years after the data are collected.[52]

In Germany, PEI acts in a similar role, aggregating data from many organizations and leading the analysis and publication of HV data. In the UK, SHOT serves in this capacity and publishes annual reports. In Japan, JRCS Blood Service Headquarters' Safety Vigilance Division aggregates HV data and publish reports. JRCS also shares data with the national MHLW and reports this information with the Pharmaceuticals and Medical Devices Agency.[53]

HV Lessons Summary

Increased participation, better reporter adherence to case definitions, and a centralized organization to aggregate, analyze, and disseminate data may all help to identify and address transfusion-related problems in the U.S. system.[54] This list of three foreign HV practices might not be exhaustive, and other HV best practices (such as efforts to apply HV to donors, not just to blood recipients) could also prove useful.

Best Practice 2: Improved Regulatory Environment for Medical Devices

Regulatory approval processes, most of which are managed by FDA under U.S. law, play a critical role in ensuring the safety of the U.S. blood system. FDA regulates the establishment of new blood centers, approves and monitors manufacturing of blood and blood products, approves devices used in the manufacturing of blood, and regulates blood products. After FDA approves a blood test, it can also require that blood establishments use particular tests to ensure blood safety—requirements that have driven, for example, the timely development and adoption of tests for HIV, West Nile virus, and Zika.

A full review of the U.S. and foreign regulatory environments is beyond the scope of this chapter, but we did examine the regulatory environment for blood-related medi-

---

[49] Wood et al., 2012; NBA, 2015a, p. 6.

[50] Australian Red Cross, "Residual Risk Estimates for Transfusion-Transmissible Infections," February 2016.

[51] Robillard, 2008, slide 37.

[52] Ditomasso, Liu, and Heddle, 2012.

[53] Okazaki, 2007.

[54] Dodd and Katz, 2015.

cal devices and associated biologic products for the countries listed in Table 9.3. These devices include items essential to the collection, processing, and transfusion of blood, such as blood bags, tubes, testing assays and equipment, and machines that collect or process blood into various products.

Our analysis of regulatory approval costs and approval procedures for such medical devices and blood additives included a review of related publications, plus interviews with FDA, blood centers, and suppliers of services and equipment. These sources indicate that the U.S. regulatory environment is one factor that slows the adoption of new technologies in the United States, especially in the current environment of low margins for blood centers and their suppliers. While some amount of cost, friction, and delay is inevitable and appropriate in any country's regulatory environment, the following data and case studies indicate that U.S. regulators could continue to incrementally apply best practices observed in several foreign countries to encourage more and faster development and adoption of improved devices and processes. It is worth noting, however, that some U.S. stakeholders have suggested that because incentives to

Table 9.3
Overview of National Regulatory Departments and Agencies for Blood and Medical Devices

Country or Region	Regulatory Authority
Australia	Therapeutic Goods Administration, national blood service (ARCBS) required to participate directly in the submission process
Canada	Health Canada's Biologics and Genetic Therapies Directorate
EU	European Council Directive 93/42/EEC requires all medical devices to meet common EU standards and use a CE Mark that is reported to national "notified bodies." Inappropriate use of the CE Mark by a manufacturer shall be reported by member states to the European Commission.
EU—Germany	After the CE Mark, PEI issues marketing authorizations, German states issue (blood) manufacturing licenses (MLs)
EU—Italy	CE Mark for devices, blood sales approved at the local level by regional health agencies or as part of a national DRG. Specific regulatory processes differ by region.[a]
EU—UK	After CE Mark, Safety of Blood Tissues and Organs is an independent review body which advises health ministers in the Department of Health and in the devolved administrations concerning blood safety measures
Japan	Pharmaceuticals and Medical Devices Agency, Pharmaceutical and Food Safety Bureau, MHLW, and JRCS are required to participate directly in the submission process
United States	FDA's CBER

SOURCES: RAND summaries based on each government's regulatory website(s) and interviews with device manufacturers.
[a] International Society for Pharmacoeconomics, "Italy—Medical Devices and Diagnostics," 2012.

invest in innovative testing and related technologies that improve the blood safety are low, many innovations are reactive to FDA mandates that tend to apply incrementally as new pathogens emerge.[55] In some sense, this increases the demands on FDA as the number of emergent pathogens threatening blood safety continues to increase. Preferences for and perceptions of FDA's role also vary across key stakeholders in the United States. For example, blood centers have conveyed to FDA that they prefer tests to perform with high sensitivity and specificity before they go on the market, which can only be demonstrated by testing in the setting of use, which imposes burdens of cost and complexity on manufacturers.

Increasing the Speed and Decreasing the Cost of Regulatory Approvals for Medical Devices

Although U.S. regulators have achieved numerous successes in protecting U.S. consumers by ensuring the safety of blood-related devices and processes, the current regulatory system is sometimes viewed as slowing or preventing the uptake of safe and effective new technologies. Several blood sector device suppliers who we interviewed voiced such concerns about the United States' regulatory approval processes for medical devices.

One device manufacturer mentioned that these concerns have become particularly worrisome in the context of falling margins on U.S. device sales. He stated that,

> We're not faulting the FDA, but their requirements are burdensome. For example, we have a product that is already approved to use for five days that we just need to get approved for seven days, but it would cost us millions of dollars to get simple approval for this and takes years, so it's not feasible. . . . Combined with FDA hurdles to jump over, and small expected returns, large companies would rather produce higher-margin products that are not blood-related.

Another blood testing device manufacturer stated that

> Regulatory requirements and costs of compliance make it very hard to invest in new technologies or even update current ones unless there is a very large market potential. These erect barriers to entry for smaller players, but also can hurt larger players as well who may not find enough return on investment after dealing with regulatory burdens.

At the same time, some blood testing manufacturers have suggested that blood centers and hospitals will not pay for innovation in testing and processing without FDA mandates. This poses a challenge for FDA, as it needs to ensure the safety of the

---

[55] Edward Snyder, Susan L. Stramer, and Richard Benjamin, "The Safety of the Blood Supply—Time to Raise the Bar," *New England Journal of Medicine*, Vol. 372, No. 20, May 14, 2015, pp. 1882–1885.

blood system but in a way that does not cause a mass exodus from the market or discourage new entry into the market.

An FDA official acknowledged that the current financial environment for blood centers and their suppliers is difficult, and that the costs of regulatory compliance are significant. However, he emphasized that the United States should not lower its regulatory standards to increase the financial incentives of bringing a new medical device to market. Instead, given the United States' substantial wealth, he argued that we could identify new sources of funding for bringing devices to market while maintaining high regulatory standards. We further explore this theme later in this chapter.

Standards across these nations are not equal, so the above data might result from the U.S. regulators enforcing higher standards. The quality of submissions to regulators might also vary, as well as the amount of time that sponsors take to respond to regulators' questions. Although several device manufacturers stated that the Emergo Group estimates track well with their experiences, FDA data specific to Class III medical devices indicate that total approval times have dropped significantly as compared with the U.S. estimates. One medical device manufacturer noted the FDA efforts, stating that "The FDA has been trying to address this by having user fees and time clocks." In 2016, an FDA/CBER official stated that "Total time to decision for Class III has come down. With a panel review, our highest recent totals were 14.6 months in 2013, and now it's 11.5 months." Although FDA has recently made progress in reducing blood-related medical device approval times, further improvements would still be required to match other nations' average approval times. Furthermore, one device manufacturer stated that he anticipates changes in the regulatory dynamics in the EU, with EU-wide device approvals (CE Mark) requiring much higher performance standards than seen in the past. If both trends continue, the international gap in approval times for complex medical devices might shrink.

An FDA manager also noted that, in some respects, it is not appropriate to compare U.S. approval times with EU approval times. One reason is that CE Mark approval is different than FDA approval. A device manufacturer agreed that "In Europe, not all devices have to go through a health authority, but some national health authorities, including Germany and the UK, request their own reviews . . . unlike the U.S. system where everything goes through the FDA." Even after a national health authority in a European country approves the device, it may only be approved for use in a small number of facilities while further research is conducted. This contrasts with the U.S. system, where FDA usually requires research on device safety and efficacy to take place before final approval is granted.

Emergo Group data also indicate that U.S. Class III medical device approval costs, including all costs associated with obtaining regulatory approval, consistently top $50,000. Every other country, except Japan, provides cheaper Class III and Class IV approval processes. A device manufacturer familiar with EU regulations explained: "At a high level, the regulations in the U.S. are more stringent [than the EU's]. To get a product approved, the expenses are higher."

Case Study No. 1: Illustrating Higher U.S. Approval Costs and Longer Approval Times—INTERCEPT for Platelets and Plasma

---

PRT for platelets and plasma has been in routine use in many nations for more than ten years, under the Cerus Corporation's brand name INTERCEPT Blood System. Although this case study covers only a single technology, and one that is complex from a regulatory viewpoint, the history of INTERCEPT's regulatory approvals in various nations could still provide some generalizable insights into the ways that advanced nations handle Class III and IV devices' regulatory approvals.

INTERCEPT platelets first received regulatory approvals in the EU, acquiring the CE Mark in 2002. France approved the technology in 2003, Germany in 2007, and FDA approval in the United States occurred in 2014. Approval does not automatically lead to acceptance, and national authorities may still require further authorizations and additional studies.

The U.S. regulatory process proved particularly complex because, while the INTERCEPT Blood System is classified as a medical device, Cerus was required to submit a Premarket Approval application to FDA's CBER for regulatory clearance of both the system (INTERCEPT Blood System) and the final blood components (INTERCEPT-treated platelets and plasma). Therefore, Cerus conducted a clinical development program in conformity with that required for a biologic and provided an extensive registration dossier for the device, toxicology for the amotosalen compound and treated blood components, manufacturing validations and controls, nonclinical studies, and clinical studies.

FDA required a pivotal, randomized controlled trial for PRT, which met its primary endpoint but, according to the summary basis of approval, did not meet all secondary end points and raised a safety concern. The evidence resulting in the initial FDA decision not to approve was discussed at a Blood Product Advisory Committee meeting that recommended additional premarketing studies. Subsequently, the data of the pivotal trial were formally reanalyzed by an independent panel and published in a peer-reviewed journal. FDA reviewed the reanalysis, as well as post-marketing safety data from European national hemovigilance systems and company-sponsored studies, and approved PRT for platelets and plasma in December 2014. The European HV data became available after 2012 and enabled FDA to make a complex risk-benefit assessment that favored approval, with a Phase 4 requirement to determine whether the safety signal observed in the Phase 3 trial was real.

After FDA approval and blood center validations, blood centers in the United States were able to manufacture INTERCEPT-treated blood components for commercial sale to hospital customers, but as is standard for any interstate sale of a manufactured blood component, each U.S. blood center must submit and receive FDA approval for a supplementary Biologics License Application (BLA) for the product, the manufacturing process, and each manufacturing facility. BLAs require additional internal process validations, and the initial application may take up to a year for FDA approval. Any blood product, conventional or pathogen-reduced, that will be sold across state lines requires the manufacturing blood center to submit and receive FDA approval of a BLA for the implementation of that specific device in that process and facility. Application review time is expected to decrease if blood centers successfully complete the necessary validation and documentation requirements of FDA master BLA protocol, developed by Cerus to facilitate this process.

In the EU, the INTERCEPT Blood System received CE Mark, and additional registrations were submitted for specific country approvals of the treated platelet and plasma components. Some EU member states accepted INTERCEPT medical devices with a CE Mark without further regulatory review. However, for all blood products, including PRT products, France, Switzerland, Germany, the UK, and to some extent, Austria, have regulatory requirements beyond the initial product CE Mark. For example, in Germany, in addition to CE Mark issuance, each blood establishment must complete the following steps for commercial production of INTERCEPT blood products:

- Obtain an ML to manufacture blood components from the individual German states (Länder).
- Submit a marketing authorization application (MAA) to PEI .
- PEI review occurs within a period of seven months to one year. Clock stops extend decision more than three months.
- Provide a risk management plan before MAA license is issued.

Unlike the example for Germany, the process is centralized in such countries as France, Switzerland, and Belgium. In Canada, where the INTERCEPT Blood System for Plasma received regulatory approval in May 2016, the regulatory pathway was similar to the the the process in the United States, albeit prolonged based on the interactions required with the device and biologics divisions of Health Canada.

Japan and Australia do not accept CE Mark or FDA approval as sufficient for regulatory approval. In both Japan and Australia, the manufacturer (e.g., Cerus) cannot unilaterally submit for regulatory approval, and the national blood service (e.g., Red Cross) must be willing to engage directly in the submission process.

Therefore, if there are political, economic, or other reasons preventing blood service engagement, the registration process for a specific new product could be delayed or put on hold.

In summary, the INTERCEPT case study, when considered alongside data provided by other manufacturers of complex devices and other evidence supplied by the Emergo Group, supports the conclusion that U.S. regulatory approvals for complex medical devices take more time and money than do similar approvals in the UK, Germany, France, Switzerland, and other parts of the EU. Faster approval of devices that meet U.S. safety standards does not guarantee faster uptake, but approval is a necessary prerequisite for uptake. After approval, FDA guidance is also a critical factor influencing uptake, but, even then, other factors can delay uptake, such as the (nonregulatory) costs of adding the device to the manufacturing and testing processes. In the case of INTERCEPT, these (nonregulatory) costs are also significant, and blood centers' cost reimbursement concerns have further slowed uptake.

The U.S. system benefits from not imposing the additional hurdle of requiring a domestic blood service to engage directly in the submission process, as observed in Australia and Japan, and Canada's system appears to be equally complex and costly. The United States' BLA process may extend the time to general availability for the product of the market by up to one year, and this delay may be especially critical in situations with epidemic emerging pathogens, such as the current Zika epidemic. In addition, because FDA views blood components collected from different blood collection platforms as separate and independent products, a complex matrix of submissions and validations could further delay the general availability of U.S. blood products. FDA has been working with industry to shorten and simplify approval processes and has made progress on this front. U.S. policymakers and regulators might wish to examine EU medical device approval processes to ascertain how to further streamline and reduce the cost of U.S. approvals while maintaining high U.S. safety standards.

Harmonizing with or Converging to Internationally Prevalent Blood Safety Standards

Even the smallest differences among countries' regulatory requirements for medical devices can necessitate multiple versions of the same device, each tailored to a specific market. Creating multiple versions of a medical device to meet regulatory requirements that are unique to the U.S. adds to product development costs, which can reduce manufacturers' expected return on investment and can sometimes prevent them from offering the device to the U.S. market. When margins were higher in the U.S. blood system, profit incentives sometimes outweighed these disincentives. However, in today's low-margin environment, there is less incentive for device manufacturers to invest in new design modifications to meet any U.S. regulatory specifications that diverge from international norms.

Two examples of U.S. regulatory divergence from international norms include the FDA sample size requirements for bacterial testing and the requirement that whole blood be quickly refrigerated after collection. FDA recognizes the importance of regulatory convergence and participates in several international forums working on this issue. One forum is the Blood Cluster, which includes the European Medicines Agency, FDA, and Health Canada, where parties are trying to reach international consensus on the science supporting regulatory standards.[56] FDA also works with the Global Harmonization Task Force,[57] which was founded in 1993 to encourage a convergence in standards and regulatory practices related to medical devices. More recently, in 2011, the International Medical Device Regulators Forum also began discussing future directions in medical device regulatory harmonization,[58] and FDA is on the management committee for this forum.[59]

In the second case study, we focus on the whole blood refrigeration requirements to illustrate how such divergences in regulatory requirements can deter manufacturers from offering new devices to the U.S. market, thereby lowering the U.S. uptake of some new technologies.

Summary of Regulatory Best Practices

Some differences between the regulatory environments in the United States and other nations might result from differences in nations' underlying legal frameworks; physical factors, such as geography or disease prevalence; or structural differences in how their health systems finance, collect, process, and use blood. These larger issues would be difficult to change, so they are not fully discussed here. In Europe, for example, blood

---

[56] European Medicines Agency, "Work Plan for the CHMP Blood Products Working Party (BPWP) for 2016," London, UK, February 2016.

[57] WHO, "Global Harmonization Task Force (GHTF)," undated-b.

[58] International Medical Device Regulators Forum, home page, undated-a.

[59] International Medical Device Regulators Forum, "About IMDRF," undated-b.

Case Study No. 2: Illustrating the Importance of Harmonization with or Convergence to International Norms—Whole Blood Automation

In the EU and in many other nations, regulators allow whole blood to remain at room temperature for up to 24 hours, which allows certain blood product manufacturing processes to occur at room temperature. Manufacturers have developed some machines that process, treat, or separate whole blood at room temperature, but they are sometimes unable to sell these machines in the United States without making substantial investments in reengineering the devices. Whole blood automation (WBA) entails processing whole blood into component parts using an enclosed, fully automatic system.

According to the vice president of a large U.S. blood center, WBA allows blood centers to manufacture blood products (components) that are more uniform in volume and composition and produces more consistent, higher-quality products. We selected this as a case study because we observed uptake of this technology in all six of our comparison nations but no uptake in the United States.

This technology was first commercialized around 2003 under the trade name OrbiSac and later released in 2007 and 2008 under the Atreus brand name. Although Atreus received EU regulatory approval (CE Mark) around 2008, only a handful of blood centers in the EU, Canada, and Latin America adopted these earlier versions of the technology, as its processing speed was generally considered to be slow and its overall value proposition costly. Some U.S. blood centers also evaluated this technology around 2008 and found that these earlier versions of the machine did not provide cost-effective improvements to their manufacturing processes. Newer versions of WBA technologies have improved processing speeds and unit costs under the brand names Reveos and TACSI WB, with Reveos receiving CE Mark in 2010 and 2011.

International uptake of Reveos and similar WBA machines has been widespread, including in all of this study's six comparison nations. However, WBA is still not used in the United States, in part because FDA usually requires that whole blood be refrigerated after collection, while the manufacturer of WBA machines deems it too expensive to engineer refrigeration into the device. According to one equipment manufacturer, this is not an isolated case. However, even if and when FDA approves devices to process whole blood for 24 hours at room temperature, this alone is no guarantee that manufacturers will bring such devices to market. Shrinking U.S. demand for blood and other cost and market considerations have kept some manufacturers from bringing new technologies to market, even when FDA approved.

The regulatory impediments to bringing WBA to the United States include more than just the FDA requirement to refrigerate whole blood. For example, a medical device manufacturer stated that, "Blood component automation creates a regulatory situation where each of the derivative blood components (red cells, platelets, and plasma) have to get approved by the FDA. The cost of the initial product approval, and the cost for each blood center to revise their manufacturing processes, and aggregated regulatory complexity, impedes uptake [in the United States]."

---

products and the devices used to make them fall under the legal precept of product and producer liability, so when HCV was transmitted by transfusion, European governments paid damages to the affected people. Other nations increasingly follow the EU lead by strengthening product liability legislation.[60] The U.S. legal system, in contrast,

---

60   FindLaw, "International Product Liability Laws," undated.

focuses more on the issue of negligence rather than product liability, which might be one factor leading to differing regulatory tolerance levels for blood device safety and risk. The U.S. classifying blood additive solutions as drugs, while the EU classifies them as devices, is another example of a structural difference among nations.

Although such structural differences might be difficult to change and the U.S. system might provide superior results in terms of safety and quality, U.S. policymakers and regulators could incrementally improve the U.S. blood system's ability to adopt improved devices by further reducing average total approval times for devices and related blood manufacturing processes and by further harmonizing or converging international regulatory requirements for devices. Additionally, U.S. regulators might wish to explore additional ways to reduce device manufacturers' total costs for regulatory approvals by simplifying requirements, further subsidizing fees, or, as we discuss in the following section, defraying some of the manufacturers' costs by increasing government investments in R&D.

Best Practice 3: Coordinating and Encouraging Investments in R&D

One essential component of any nation's blood system is a healthy level of investment in R&D for processes or technologies that improve blood collection, testing, manufacturing, or transfusion. In the United States, blood centers and medical device manufacturers have historically financed and performed a significant portion of this R&D, while NIH, HHS, and DoD have financed the lion's share of blood-related R&D in the United States. However, the recent decline in profit margins for U.S. blood centers and their suppliers has led to declines in supplier-funded and blood center–funded R&D. For example, one manager of a blood test supplier stated, "From the company perspective, declining prices do not encourage research and development into new products." Another manager of a device manufacturer predicted that

> R&D could dry up based on this current situation. It's already come to the point where you don't see much innovation in this field. For example, pathogen reduction has been around 20 years but is only ramping up now. It wouldn't have been developed if R&D had to begin today.

A third manager of a supplier to the U.S. blood system stated that

> Investment by companies has pretty much stopped. For example, the companies that develop tests [e.g., tests for Dengue, Chikungunya, and Zika] have no incentive to be innovative and develop new tests because they know they can't make money and because it won't be taken up unless the FDA mandates it. Innovation is almost nonexistent.

Some managers of U.S. blood centers expressed similar concerns, while others explained why their R&D budgets are more secure. One manager of a blood center with a national presence stated that since 2007 his

> . . .R&D budget has shrunk every year . . . the most massive cuts have come in the last five or six years. Our budget has been cut more than 50 percent since its peak . . . blood centers can no longer afford to support doing research, and we can't charge for research nor make enough margin to make up for it.

However, some other blood-focused R&D centers rely on more diversified sources of revenue, including foundations with patent revenues or philanthropic donors, and others rely on NIH grants.

U.S. Government Providing Critical Support to Blood Sector R&D

As U.S. blood centers' and suppliers' R&D investments continue at lower-than-historical levels, government support for R&D has become increasingly important to maintaining the pace of innovation in the blood sector. NIH's NHLBI grants have historically been the primary vehicle for U.S. government R&D funding in the blood sector, totaling more than $400 million during FY 2012.[61] Some R&D institutes run by blood centers rely primarily on these NIH grants. NIH also provided early funding for device manufacturers' PRT, for example, and DoD has funded more than $32 million of development for PRT.

Additionally, during the past two years, HHS' ASPR, BARDA, began to invest in private corporations' research in PR and Zika testing. BARDA has historically focused on threats not related to blood production, such as medical countermeasures for pandemics and influenza, and for chemical, biological, radiological, and nuclear threats, but it has recently expanded to emerging infectious diseases. BARDA taps two funding streams (Advanced R&D and Project Bio Shield) and receives supplemental funding tied to particular issues. BARDA could increasingly serve as a critical vehicle for U.S. government support to blood sector R&D.

Advantages of Closer Coordination Among Blood Centers and Government Funders

Although the volume of money invested in U.S. blood sector R&D far outpaces levels seen in other foreign countries, other nations' R&D investment practices still yield potentially useful lessons. Namely, because some countries support blood sector R&D by running their own blood-focused research centers, they demonstrate several potential best practices, including a reduction in the duplication of effort and a more systematic ability to ascertain the cost-effectiveness and utility of R&D investments. This contrasts with the U.S. system, where blood centers play a declining role in shaping R&D priorities, while the primary sources of R&D funding are government orga-

---

[61]   NHLBI, 2012.

nizations that are somewhat disconnected from the practical implementation of blood collection, processing, and transfusion. On the plus side, this disconnect between funders and blood centers gives researchers the freedom to pursue investments in basic science that might disrupt current business practices—for example, NHLBI-funded researchers have made discoveries that could eventually revolutionize the blood sector through "blood farming."[62] However, in the short term, such research investments might not address the priorities currently facing blood centers and hospitals. Without strong linkages to the practical needs of blood sector practitioners, many R&D investments might fail to produce useful results.

While some U.S. blood centers report that a lack of coordination among U.S. research organizations results in much duplication of effort, other nations have centralized their R&D efforts under a government-run entity closely linked to their blood collection organizations. In Canada, for example, CBS's Centre for Innovation facilitates the creation, translation, and application of new knowledge to support Canada's blood system. The Centre's integration with CBS's core operations provides opportunities for cross-fertilization to enhance the efficiency and cost-effectiveness of the blood system. These activities promote the creation of new knowledge and its translation into enhanced and new practices, services, and technologies. Similar to how many U.S. blood centers offer professional training to hospital staff, Canada's Centre for Innovation formally trains professionals through its national training program.[63] Canada's Héma-Québec also runs its own R&D financing program,[64] which utilizes 5 percent of the organization's overall budget and coordinates closely with the overall objectives of its other operations. Héma-Québec's R&D Division states that one of its goals is to foster the growth of an economic environment that is favorable to innovation, highlighting the connection between R&D investments and the ability of device manufacturers to innovate.

In Australia, ARCBS obtains block funding for R&D, and special development projects are specifically funded. Again, we observe a centralized coordination of national R&D efforts via NBA. Similarly, in England, NHSBT receives grants and contributions from the British Department of Health for research. Strategic investments are funded through additional funding requests to the British Department of Health and must be supported by a business case that clearly demonstrates the benefits of the investment in terms of patient outcomes, efficiencies, and other beneficial impacts. These business cases include the investment requirements, as well as the impact to operational costs and the base-funding budget.

---

[62] Lilian Varricchio and Anna Rita Migliaccio, "The Role of Glucocorticoid Receptor (GR) Polymorphisms in Human Erythropoiesis," *American Journal of Blood Research*, Vol. 4, No. 2, 2014, p. 53.

[63] Canadian Blood Services, *Centre for Innovation Progress Report 2014–2015*, Ottawa, Canada: Centre for Innovation, June 29, 2015, p. 3.

[64] Héma-Québec, "Research and Development at Héma-Québec: An Overview," 2014.

These foreign organizations' ability to closely coordinate R&D priorities with blood centers, their ability to minimize duplication of effort across national R&D organizations, their ability to prioritize R&D efforts based on expected returns, and their closer alignment with the practical needs of blood centers are all practices that U.S. policymakers might wish to implement or encourage within the U.S. blood system. Already the United States has some ability to coordinate federally funded R&D investments via interagency committees, but given the significant amount of R&D that is not federally funded, and given the bureaucratic leeway that each U.S. agency and department has to direct funds, U.S. coordination of R&D efforts is not as advanced as witnessed in some foreign nations. As U.S. blood centers and their suppliers invest less in R&D, the importance of government-funded R&D is rising, and this could provide new opportunities to increase coordination of and prioritization of U.S. R&D efforts across the blood sector.

Conclusions and Other Best Practices

In this chapter, we focused on three broad areas in which the United States might be able to incrementally apply foreign best practices: HV, medical device regulation, and government coordination of R&D. Improvements in these three areas have the potential to improve the sustainability of the U.S. blood system, as HV systems strengthen the ability to identify and address adverse transfusion-related events, improved medical device regulation increases suppliers' incentives to innovate and deliver improved products and devices, and improved coordination of R&D investments reduces duplication of effort and increases cost-effective innovation in the blood sector.

These three best practices, however, are by no means the only ones that U.S. policymakers should consider applying here. Some other possible candidates that we were not able to fully address include

- the possibility of subsidizing blood manufacturing, processing, or testing, as witnessed in many foreign nations, including Canada, Australia, and the UK
- the advantages of combining blood center operations with other operations, such as collection and testing for tissues, organs, cord blood, and more. Some U.S. blood centers, such as VERSITI, have already identified synergies from testing blood and organs in the same facilities, for example. However, in other countries, such as Canada, we witnessed the national blood centers participating in sectors beyond blood
- the deregulation of apheresis plasma originally collected for transfusion into sales to fractionators. In the United States, apheresis plasma collected for transfusion cannot be sold to fractionators until it has expired (one year after collection).

CHAPTER TEN

Conclusion: Themes and Recommendations

In this final chapter, we provide a synthesis of the preceding chapters with three main objectives. First, we highlight overarching and shared themes that emerged across multiple research questions and earlier chapters. Second, we propose a set of recommendations to promote a sustainable U.S. blood system informed by our study for both policymakers and stakeholders more broadly. Finally, we discuss the limitations of our study and next steps for research in this area.

Key Themes

The bolded themes in this section are informed by our work mainly in Chapters Four through Nine, with many themes drawing on insights and findings from multiple chapters. The themes are organized in groups: (1) overarching findings, (2) specific implications of threats to sustainability, and (3) opportunities to improve sustainability. Each theme listed is accompanied by a short description and justification.

Overarching Findings
The U.S. blood system under the status quo operates effectively and, in many cases, efficiently. Although our report focuses on challenges related to blood system sustainability, it is important to recognize the success of the system under the status quo. Overall, we found that blood was always or almost always available to hospitals. Stakeholders—including blood centers in particular—relocate units to minimize outdating and wastage and to respond to a range of unanticipated needs. Finally, robust price competition controls blood costs.

  The U.S. blood system is in a period of flux and uncertainty. Chapter Four lays out some of the most important perceived internal trends and external pressures facing the blood system, and particularly blood centers, including a marked decrease in demand for blood, rising imbalance between buyer power and seller power in blood markets, and increasing safety standards and associated production costs. These financial pressures on blood centers might affect the sustainability of the blood system if they result in significant and sudden changes in supply that cannot be addressed with available surge capacity. Such pressures may be particularly problematic for local or regional blood centers that are less likely to have the ability to offset losses in one market with gains from another market or another line of business. However, the blood system has over time responded to a wide range of profound technological, clinical, and policy changes. Current pressures and trends might serve as a catalyst for innovation and evolution in the blood system for at least some stakeholders.

There are unlikely but possible scenarios in which the supply of blood would be disrupted. As is the case with many other inputs into the production of health care services—including drugs, devices, and professional services—disruptions in supply can affect the timing and type of care delivered to patients, potentially with important implications for health outcomes and health care spending. Chapter Nine describes the risks from a range of scenarios. As with other parts of the health care system, a major event or disaster or a combination of multiple smaller events could lead to shortages of blood. It is difficult to gauge whether the system has sufficient surge capability to respond to the most serious events.

Specific Implications of Threats to Sustainability

The current system is not conducive to private investments in innovation. Blood centers, their suppliers, and the government invest in R&D with the potential to improve the U.S. blood system. Shrinking profit margins to blood centers coupled with generally weak business cases for the purchasers of blood to pay for some new technologies limit the current extent of private investment in innovation. The current investment decisions of blood centers and their suppliers depend somewhat precariously on the financial stability of linked nodes in the supply chain. Thus, if blood centers are unable to pass on costs of innovation to hospitals, this affects not only blood centers but also other firms' willingness to invest in new innovation. This could potentially have serious consequences for the safety and sustainability of the U.S. blood system.

Suppliers to blood centers face significant uncertainty and contribute to concerns about sustainability. Suppliers of equipment, products, and services that are necessary inputs into the U.S. blood system face financial pressures spilling over from blood centers. In many cases, there is one supplier or a small number of suppliers for specific inputs—for example, filters used in blood collection. Large suppliers exiting the blood sector could cause substantial disruption to the U.S. blood system, as regulatory and other barriers to entry complicate rapid entry by other firms.

Services provided by local blood banks may be at risk. Both hospitals and blood centers placed significant value on having local partners—in part to ensure rapid access to a supply of blood and in part because of collaboration and services shared between stakeholders. In interviews, many stakeholders noted the importance of local relationships, citing such benefits as the training that blood center experts provide to hospital transfusion staff and the speed at which community blood banks can meet the evolving needs of hospitals. However, as the market for blood has become increasingly national in scope and hospitals are consolidating into large systems at a rapid pace, there are concerns that these community-based links between hospitals and blood centers are at risk. Despite the frequent mention of the benefits offered by local partners, there is nothing preventing blood centers with national scope from offering similar services or support.

Opportunities to Improve Sustainability

Stakeholders want support in making technology adoption decisions. Maintaining safety is an integral feature of the U.S. blood system. Regulators tasked with ensuring the safety of the blood supply—including CDC, FDA, NIH, and other components of HHS—face threats that can sometimes be addressed by adopting existing technology. However, decisions regarding the adoption of innovations that will increase production costs (such as a Zika virus test) or address threats more broadly (such as PRT) are especially challenging for blood centers, given information asymmetries and the current financial environment. In some cases, technology adoption is mandated by FDA or has become the industry standard. In other cases, individual blood centers and hospitals make decisions about what technology to adopt and what products to buy. Our stakeholder interviews suggest that not all blood centers and hospitals feel equipped to make these decisions; there are uncertainties with respect to which technologies will be approved by FDA (if required) and which ones will be cost-effective. A robust conversation on the cost-effectiveness of these technologies from the stakeholder and societal perspective and patients' preferences could help guide HHS policymaking in this area, as well as private decisionmaking.

Blood center stakeholders are contemplating different market structures for the future. Many blood center stakeholders spoke in general terms about the potential for consolidation among blood centers, a more substantial government role in ensuring an adequate supply of blood, and the changing dynamics between ARC and independent blood centers. That blood center stakeholders are identifying and evaluating alternate structures and arrangements in their industry is a sign that the private sector might ultimately address some of the key threats to sustainability without government intervention. At the same time, new players, including brokerages, are introducing new technology and services that might catalyze additional changes. These changes might not preclude the potential role for government intervention in certain areas of the market, as, for example, with involvement with investment in mandated testing or other areas where there may be market failure.

All stakeholders recognize the important role of blood as a public health good. This recognition includes the importance of available blood for routine and unexpected health care services and for use in responding to emergency events. While there was agreement on the importance of surge capacity in general, stakeholders had different opinions on the ability of the current system to continue to meet these demands, although the system has largely been able to meet emergency needs to date.

Broad Alternatives for the Future of the Blood System

Together, these themes describe a blood system currently achieving its objectives in terms of supply but with risks to its future sustainability. Our report outlines a variety of pressures on blood centers and their suppliers, including decreasing demand for blood, falling unit prices, increasing buyer power, payment policies that do not directly reflect the use of blood, and new safety concerns and regulatory requirements. Some of these pressures—for example, decreasing demand for blood and falling unit prices— are positive developments from the perspective of patients, providers, and policymakers. One important, common driver of these pressures is a fundamental imbalance in the market for blood, where hospital buyers have significant leverage in negotiations, many blood center suppliers offering similar products have little power, and there has been no change over time in the number of blood centers despite the significant decline in demand. The most common pressures cited by blood centers stem from these market conditions. If there were more of a balance between buyers and sellers, blood centers would presumably be able to charge higher prices.

A desire on the part of blood centers to improve their market position is not itself a rationale for policy action. However, if the pressures facing blood centers lead to unexpected or rapid changes in the supply of blood—for example, as a result of a wave of blood center closures—policy could help minimize the negative consequences from these changes. Furthermore, the negative externalities from the status quo blood system—including a lack of private resources to invest in technology and innovation— may not be desirable from the societal perspective.

One broad alternative is to let the U.S. blood system continue to function as it has without new policy intervention, with private organizations (including blood centers and hospitals) making key decisions on production and utilization facilitated by current levels of government regulation and intervention. Overall, we expect that this approach will continue to result in a safe, sustainable blood system. Given current market conditions, we expect that blood centers will consolidate over time without government intervention, improving the balance between supply and demand for blood in terms of volume and negotiating power. However, there are several potential significant risks under the status quo, particularly if suppliers of blood consolidate quickly or unpredictably in response to market pressures. Although allowing the market to adjust naturally may yield a market equilibrium that is more stable in the long term, such adjustments might negatively affect other aspects of the system in the short term (e.g., loss of surge capacity and temporary shortages).

Another broad alternative is for the government to take a more active role in regulating or supporting the blood system—for example, by collecting more data for analysis and monitoring; adjusting how private and public health insurers pay for blood and health care services involving blood; and paying explicitly for certain technologies or features of the blood system, such as tests and surge capacity, where there is a clear public good or spillover justification for the funding. An expansion of the government's role in the U.S. blood system also carries risks, such as the introduction of market distortions that could raise the overall cost of delivering blood, but it could be justified on the grounds that blood is a public health good requiring nonmarket interventions to optimize quality and reliability.

A third broad alternative is for the government to assume complete responsibility for the supply of blood, mirroring the government-operated blood systems in other countries, such as the UK. This approach would be a major departure from the status quo and could remove or weaken the system's current incentives to reduce costs. On the other hand, this approach would let policymakers manage routine supply and surge capacity that fit with the needs of the health care system and with public health.

We do not see the justification for a transition to an entirely public blood system in the United States. This transition would be very disruptive—perhaps more so than the first alternative in which blood centers and hospitals continue under the status quo. Instead, we propose that the middle broad alternative in terms of policy intervention—in which the blood system remains privatized but with some additional government intervention—balances benefits from opportunities to improve sustainability against the risks and frictional costs from wholesale changes to the system. Under this approach, the government's role would be to ensure the sustainability of the current blood system. Some aspects of the current system—for example, price competition between blood centers—are meeting some policy objectives (i.e., limiting the contribution of blood to health care spending growth). Rather than completely replacing functioning aspects of this industry and accompanying incentive structures, we propose a set of narrower recommendations that HHS could consider to improve blood system sustainability. Our recommendations in the following section are all in the vein of incremental government intervention supporting a continued private market for blood.

Recommendations

In this section, we outline several recommendations for consideration to improve the sustainability of the U.S. blood system. These seven recommendations could be implemented separately or in conjunction with one another. Some of the recommendations—for example, subsidies to blood centers—might require statutory changes to implement, while others—for example, building a blood "safety net"—fall within the current HHS authority. Several recommendations suggested to RAND researchers from stakeholders throughout the project are not on our final list of recommendations to HHS, including a blood pass-through in Medicare payment policy. In this specific case, a combination of other recommendations—including the recommendation for data collection on blood utilization, prices, and costs and the recommendation for specific payments to blood centers for maintaining surge capacity and adopting new technologies—address the key underlying issues that led to the discussion on a blood pass-through. Furthermore, the likely effects of a pass-through depend on how the policy is designed in terms of payment rates and other features.

Recommendation 1: Collect data on blood use and financial arrangements. While stakeholders have access to statistics on blood use and transactions related to their individual organizations, the government currently does not have access to comprehensive data describing the performance of the blood system as a whole. Based on our review of available data, NBCUS currently offers the most comprehensive view into blood utilization and prices. However, this survey is relatively small in terms of sample size (particularly for hospitals), has a modest response rate, and does not capture granular data on individual transactions or uses. While hospitals report detailed utilization data to Medicare on an ongoing basis to update payment rates, stakeholders reported that these data are often incomplete and cover only Medicare patients. HHS should conduct ongoing time and motion studies to clarify how blood is used in different settings. In addition, HHS could require reporting of blood volume and payment rate data as a requirement for participation in surge capacity or technology adoption programs (described in Recommendations 3 and 6). These data would allow for analyses of physician-patient–level blood utilization, whereas NBCUS data contain aggregated hospital or blood center–level data.

Recommendation 2: Develop and disseminate a vision for appropriate levels of surge capacity and emergency response plans. Despite universal recognition among stakeholders of the importance of surge capacity, no stakeholder was able to articulate exactly what level of capacity was sufficient or optimal. Although we heard from stakeholders and found some evidence that a three- to seven-day supply is considered sufficient (see discussion in Chapter Six), this measure does not translate easily into a systemwide surge capacity measure. For example, there is variation in how many units of blood constitute a one-day supply, as this tends to be based on a given hospital or blood center's level of activity. Additionally, as pointed out in most retrospective assessments of blood demands in past public health emergencies, blood on the shelf is what is used in emergencies, not blood collected during emergencies (although collections during emergencies are also necessary to replenish available supply). Thus, policymakers and the blood system would benefit from a clearer understanding of how to quantify system-wide surge capacity. HHS should conduct a needs assessment study to characterize the specific features and functionality of a U.S. blood system with appropriate surge capacity. Clearly describing the desired level of surge capacity from a public health and preparedness perspective will help isolate the related costs to the system from the usual transaction-based arrangements between blood centers and hospitals.

Recommendation 3: Pay blood centers for maintaining surge capacity. The motivation for this recommendation is from two sources. First, surge capacity to respond to serious events and emergencies falls outside the typical financial arrangements between hospitals and blood centers. In the current environment of falling demand for blood and resulting excess supply, centers have shown some surge capacity to meet emergency needs, such as the demand for blood shipments to Puerto Rico because of the Zika virus crisis. However, once the industry has adjusted to lower demand in Puerto Rico, there is no guarantee that this surge capacity will remain. If blood centers are asked to retain excess staff, collection capabilities, or stock for any reason other than the current demand for blood from hospitals, there is a strong argument that the government should separately finance this surge capacity. Second, financial pressures from an increasingly national market for blood place some local blood centers at a disadvantage relative to large, national centers, such as ARC.

The government could finance blood surge capacity through grants similar to those awarded by HRSA to FQHCs. The magnitude of the payments should be calibrated to incentivize blood centers to maintain particular levels of surge capacity (in terms of labor, equipment, space, donor base, supply, and more) relative to their total volume of collections or number of hospitals or markets served. Receipt of funding could be tied to accountability provisions, including review of arrangements between the blood center and hospitals or emergency response plans (see Recommendation 2).

Recommendation 4: Build relationships with brokers and other entities to form a blood "safety net." HHS recently intervened to facilitate the delivery of blood to Puerto Rico in response to the Zika virus crisis through an arrangement with ARC. HHS should build ongoing relationships with ARC, ASBP, and brokerage entities (e.g., Bloodbuy). These entities would commit to procuring and delivering blood at the request of HHS to address short-term and local shortages. While a blood safety net provides some assurance of a timely, safe, and adequate supply of blood in the case of emergency events, it can also help smooth short-term, localized disruptions in supply caused by consolidation among blood centers or other market changes. In terms of implementation, the government could bear the transactional costs of setting up and maintaining the network and transporting product, while per unit payments are treated differently depending on whether the need for the safety net supply is due to an emergency event or another event, such as the exit of a blood center from a market. In the former case, the government could decide to pay the per-unit costs, while in the latter case, hospital purchasers could pay per-unit rates—perhaps at the same prices that they had been paying to their past providers.

Recommendation 5: Build and implement a value framework for new technology. In many cases that we reviewed in the literature and discussed with stakeholders, the benefits from new technologies (including pathogen-specific tests and broader PRTs) simply do not justify their cost from the perspective of a hospital buyer. However, from the broader societal perspective, where concerns on safety and sustainability are paramount, these interventions might make sense even without a business case from the hospital or blood centers' point of view. In this scenario, however, adoption rates will be low without government intervention through mandates or financing. Our recommendation is for HHS to invest in health technology assessment research for existing technologies with low adoption rates (for example, PRTs) and technologies on the horizon. These analyses should distinguish between costs and benefits accruing to blood centers and hospitals and costs and benefits from the broader societal perspective. They should also assess the extent to which certain technologies may preclude the need for testing or other processing (e.g., PR might make testing for certain agents unnecessary), which has implications for investments in those technologies. For technologies with significant costs and benefits from the societal perspective but not from the blood center and hospital perspectives, other policy intervention could encourage adoption.

Recommendation 6: Pay directly for new technologies where there is no private business case for adoption. As noted in the description of Recommendation 5, decisions to broadly adopt some tests (e.g., babesia) that are now industry standards are difficult to justify from the business perspectives of blood centers and hospitals. However, these technologies often have clear public health and preparedness benefits, and policymakers might want to require or at least encourage adoption. In these cases, government financing of technology acquisition costs may be appropriate. One possibility would be to use BARDA's procurement authority to acquire technologies under the recommendation of the secretary of HHS that are integral to public health (e.g., a Zika virus screening test). Government subsidies for technology adoption could also target interoperable IT infrastructure specific to blood.

Recommendation 7: Implement emergency use authorization and contingency planning for key supplies and inputs. In addition to preparing for emergencies or unexpected events that affect the supply and demand for blood, HHS should consider regulatory pathways to address shortages of key supplies and inputs for the blood system. Supply manufacturers have noted that market incentives to remain in the blood sector are sometimes weak, and that, should a supplier decide to exit the market for blood-related products, it could take months for another supplier to ramp up production of the product. The recent recall of filters used in leukoreduction also highlights the important role of suppliers in the sustainability of the blood system.[1] HHS could—through FDA—implement emergency use authorizations for replacement supplies and other inputs in the event of a shortage. More broadly, FDA and HHS should engage in a dialogue with suppliers on regulatory approval requirements and expectations.

Limitations and Knowledge Gaps

We did not have access to systematic data on the transactions between hospitals and blood centers, and we were unable to access the response-level NBCUS data. As a result,

---

[1] FDA, "Urgent Recall Extension for Leukotrap RC System with RC2D Filter," press release, June 20, 2016c.

we used available aggregated data from the peer-reviewed literature, prior NBCUS reports, CMS, and FDA. Our first recommendation outlines a rationale for the collection of more-robust and representative data on how blood is donated, used, and paid for in the U.S. blood system. Richer data will facilitate empirical analyses on blood markets and the blood system that were not possible in the current study.

Our qualitative data collection effort involved conversations with ten blood center representatives, eight hospital representatives, eight suppliers to blood centers, and a range of government and nongovernment experts. While our qualitative interviews included all major stakeholder groups, we spoke to relatively few individuals in each group. In order to mitigate this limitation, at the end of our study, we separately spoke to current and former HHS blood experts, as well an external peer reviewer who was able to provide a high-level confirmation that the information we collected through our conversations was generalizable.

Throughout much of the report, we assumed that blood collection, the processing technology, and the use of blood in clinical practice would remain relatively constant over the next decade. We noted that some stakeholders predict greater declines in blood utilization in the future, which could have implications for our recommendations, depending on the magnitude of the decline. We did not model future blood utilization, and thus our analysis and recommendations are based largely on the decline noted to date. Although we discuss some aspects of technological disruptions to the system, there are other, more-radical changes on the longer-term horizon with varying degrees of likelihood, such as artificial blood or blood farming. These technologies have the potential to completely reshape the blood system in such a way that our analyses and recommendations would no longer apply.

Interview Protocols

Interview Protocol for Blood Centers

Informed consent: RAND is working in consultation with HHS to describe and analyze the U.S. blood system. Today's interview will focus on the blood centers' perspective on challenges and opportunities in the U.S. blood supply as well as the role of your organization in the supply chain including management, use, and payment for blood products. The discussion of our meeting will be kept confidential. RAND staff will be taking notes during the meeting, but only summary information from the meeting will be included in our final report. We will not identify a specific individual by name or affiliation without his or her permission.

Although documents related to this project may reveal who participated in these interviews, your responses and ideas will be combined with others and reported in a group. Your participation in this interview is entirely voluntary. You do not have to participate in the interview, and if you participate, you should feel free to skip any questions. We believe the risks to participation are minimal. Do you have any questions about our confidentiality procedures before we begin? (If yes, respond to all questions. If no, proceed with discussion.)

Introduction

1. Please describe your role in your blood center as well as specifics related to your role in the collection and management of blood at your center?
2. Thank you for having emailed to us some basic statistics on your blood center (e.g., your affiliations and partnerships, location(s), volumes of blood collected, etc.).
   a. Alternate: If interviewee has not yet shared this information that RAND requested via email, RAND can remind them to please send it.
3. Please describe other blood centers in your local area. Do other blood centers supply hospitals in your community/region? Do they sometimes supply the same hospitals that you supply?

How Your Center Works—From Blood Drives to Blood Delivery

1. Does your organization organize and/or hold blood drives? If yes, please describe (e.g., number, frequency, etc.).
    a. Does your center (or any centers) ever turn away donors when donations surge or stocks are high?
2. How does your blood center screen donors before they give blood, or to target donors who are ideal for giving blood?
    a. Would you be willing to share a copy of your screening questionnaire with us?
3. Your blood center emailed RAND that it collects ___ units of RBC per year and ___ units of platelets per year. Does this vary by time of year/season? Have you been expanding collections or reducing collections during the past 3 years?
    a. If they have not yet answered RAND's emailed request for volumes of blood collected, remind them to please do so.
4. After a unit of blood is collected, what typically happens to that blood before it is delivered to a hospital for use? Which parts of this process happen internally?
    a. To what extent is blood testing and processing performed by your organization?
    b. What blood tests and/or blood processing procedures are performed by third parties that are not blood centers nor hospitals?
    c. Later in this interview, we'll ask some questions about the costs of each of these steps.
5. Does your blood center have relationships in place to obtain blood from other suppliers when you are unable to supply a sufficient quantity, or do you leave that to the hospitals to prepare backup plans?
6. How is the blood stored and transported either to testing/processing facilities or hospitals?
    a. How do you track what you have (capture and define stock levels)?
    b. How do you forecast demand for blood?
7. Thank you for sharing via email how many hospital blood banks you supply blood to. How often do you receive blood requests from these customers? What is the frequency of your blood deliveries? What are the processes involved in ordering blood? What triggers an order?
    a. If they did not yet answer RAND's email request for information on the hospitals they supply, RAND can remind them to please do so.
8. Are there any principles/general practices that you apply to blood management, such as first in first out? Please describe. What polices/programs do you have in place to reduce waste/outdating?

a. Do you use any software/systems, equipment, and/or tools to manage your blood collection and stock? Please describe.

Contract Costs and Payments

1. We are interested in learning about the contractual arrangements blood centers make with hospitals/providers. Can you tell us what terms are typically included in these agreements?

   a. What is the frequency of delivery, volume of blood that must be stocked?

   b. Who handles/pays for blood inventory management?

   c. Are transportation, storage, testing, and other costs individually itemized and charged to the hospitals, or do hospitals pay one lump sum per unit which may or may not include all of these logistical costs?

   d. What is the cost of a unit of blood?
      ◦ Could you share any data or estimates of what cost components go into the total cost of blood?
      ◦ How does this cost vary over time (season variation or trends)?
      ◦ Does it vary across types (is AB worth more than O+ , etc.)?
      ◦ Are there different prices for units based on its freshness upon delivery?

   e. When do blood centers receive payment for blood—is it only based on the volumes of blood transfused, or based on volumes ordered and delivered?
      ◦ Probe: In general terms, what is the structure of payment arrangements between your organization and hospitals? A single payment per unit time? Per-unit payment? Some combination of the two? Something else?

   f. How would your contractual arrangements with hospitals change if the FDA were to require pathogen reduction (PR)?
      ◦ Prompt if needed: Would you negotiate new payment rates?
      ◦ What factors led you to invest in (or not invest in) pathogen reduction (PR) and other safety testing or processing that goes beyond what is FDA-required? How do such investments affect your center's financial bottom line?

   g. Do you feel that your organization is adequately compensated for blood delivered from your center? Why or why not? Do you have concerns about this going forward in the future?
      ◦ Probe: Are you pleased with the contract arrangements you have with your blood consumers? Are there any problems? What works well? Are there any changes you could think of that would improve the contracts?

Health Care System Trends

1. What trends/developments on the horizon in the health care system concern you? Have the potential to negatively impact your business?
    a. Probe on affordable care organizations, global payments, ACA coverage expansion, medical device excise tax, consolidation of hospital markets.
    b. Do you have any plans to make changes (e.g., business practices) to address these threats? If yes, please describe. What about your industry more broadly—are others making changes?
2. What trends/developments in the health care system are you excited about? Have the potential to positively impact your business?
    a. Probe on affordable care organizations, global payments, ACA coverage expansion, medical device excise tax, consolidation of hospital markets.
    b. Do you have any plans to make changes (e.g., business practices) to take better advantage of these opportunities? If yes, please describe. What about your industry more broadly—are others making changes?
3. We are thinking about how to improve the U.S blood supply chain from vein to vein. Do you have any concerns about the sustainability of the system as it currently exists or any recommendations to improve how blood is managed?
4. Is there anything you would like to add that we did not discuss today?
5. Are there others at your center who have detailed knowledge of the issues that we discussed that we should talk to?

Interview Protocol for Hospitals

Informed consent: RAND is working in consultation with HHS to describe and analyze the U.S. blood system. Today's interview will focus on the hospital perspective on challenges and opportunities in the U.S. blood supply as well as the role of your organization in the supply chain including management, use, and payment for blood products. The discussion of our meeting will be kept confidential. RAND staff will be taking notes during the meeting, but only summary information from the meeting will be included in our final report. We will not identify a specific individual by name or affiliation without his or her permission.

Although documents related to this project may reveal who participated in these interviews, your responses and ideas will be combined with others and reported in a group. Your participation in this interview is entirely voluntary. You do not have to participate in the interview, and if you participate, you should feel free to skip any questions. We believe the risks to participation are minimal. Do you have any questions about our confidentiality procedures before we begin? (If yes, respond to all questions. If no, proceed with discussion.)

Questions for all Hospital Interviews

Introduction

1. Please describe your role in your hospital as well as specifics related to your role in the management and use of blood at your hospital.
2. Please briefly describe your hospital (e.g., number of beds, teaching vs. not).

Inventory

1. How much blood (and what kinds of blood products) do you store at your hospital at any given time?
2. How do you track what you have (capture and define stock levels)? Do you use any tools/software to help with this? Do the blood banks help with this?
3. If you use any software solutions to manage blood inventory, what functions does it fulfill and what other functionality would be beneficial for blood inventory management?
4. How do you forecast demand for blood?
5. Who (and how many blood banks) supply blood to you? How often do you receive blood from these suppliers/frequency of deliveries? What are the processes involved in ordering to replenish depleted stocks? What triggers an order?
6. Are you pleased with the contract/arrangements/relationships you have with your suppliers? Are there any problems?
7. Are there any principles/general practices that you apply to blood management such as first in first out? Please describe.
8. What polices/programs do you have in place to reduce waste/outdating? How frequently does waste occur (or roughly what percent of all blood is wasted)?
9. Do you use any software/systems, equipment, and/or tools to manage your blood stock? Please describe.
10. How are specific units allocated to patients? Is there any internal coordinating of scheduling of procedures that might potentially use blood and current blood stock?
11. Where is blood stored? Do you have dedicated staff or systems to manage temperature and storage conditions? Have you ever had to discard blood due to inadequate or compromised storage conditions?

Internal vs. External Processes

1. Roughly what percent of the blood (allogeneic) in your stock do you collect at your hospital? Do you also do autologous blood transfusions? What proportion of all transfusions are autologous?
2. If you collect blood at your hospital, do you perform all testing and processing of that internally collected blood, or does internally collected blood ever leave

the hospital premises for testing or processing? How does this vary when autologous vs. allogenic?

3. When blood arrives at your hospital from an external source, what testing and processing has already been performed by external organizations, and what testing and/or processing remains to be done at your hospital?

Use

1. Do you have a patient blood management program at your facility? If yes, please explain what it involves. Has it been successful at reducing the number of transfusions/number of units transfused? (If not, do you have any systems, programs, policies, etc. in place to reduce demand for transfusions? Please describe.)

2. Does your hospital experience blood shortages? How often are standard/routine orders incomplete? What is the impact of a shortage on the hospital (e.g., canceled elective surgeries)? What do you do in response to shortages?

Overall

1. We are thinking about how to improve the U.S blood supply chain from vein to vein. Do you have any concerns about the sustainability of the system as it currently exists? Any recommendations to improve how blood is managed at any stage of the process?

2. Anything you would like to add that we did not discuss today?

3. Are there others at your facility who have detailed knowledge of the issues that we discussed that we should talk to?

Additional Questions for Hospital Managers/Finance Specialists Only

Payment

1. Are transfusions at your hospital adequately reimbursed? Why or why not?

2. We understand that for Medicare, hospital costs (paying for blood, managing inventory, cross-matching, etc) are rolled into the DRG, so you are not paid separately for blood. Is this the case with other payers? How does reimbursement work for the private payers and Medicaid at your hospital?

3. Do you face any challenges in billing and being reimbursed for blood transfusions?

Interview Protocols for Suppliers, Regulators, and Other Blood Sector Experts

RAND did not develop a separate, formal protocol for these populations. Rather, we adapted the blood center and hospital protocols on a case-by-case basis. Therefore, interviews with suppliers, regulators, and other blood sector experts were not as uniformly structured as were the blood center and hospital interviews.

Bibliography

AABB—*See* American Association of Blood Banks.

ABC—*See* America's Blood Centers.

Adams, Sophie, Florent Baarsch, Alberte Bondeau, Dim Coumou, Reik Donner, Katja Frieler, Bill Hare, Arathy Menon, Mahe Perette, Franziska Piontek, Kira Rehfeld, Alexander Robinson, Marcia Rocha, Joeri Rogelj, Jakob Runge, Michiel Schaeffer, Jacob Schewe, Carl-Friedrich Schleussner, Susanne Schwan, Olivia Serdeczny, Anastasia Svirejeva-Hopkins, Marion Vieweg, Lila Warszawski, and World Bank, *Turn Down the Heat: Climate Extremes, Regional Impacts, and the Case for Resilience—Full Report*, Washington, D.C.: World Bank, 2013. As of October 18, 2016:
http://documents.worldbank.org/curated/en/975911468163736818/
Turn-down-the-heat-climate-extremes-regional-impacts-and-the-case-for-resilience-full-report

Adams, Steve, "Health Reform to Leave Its Mark; Consumers, Businesses, Biotech May Benefit in Massachusetts," *The Patriot Ledger*, March 27, 2010.

Alter, Harvey J., Susan L. Stramer, and Roger Y. Dodd, "Emerging Infectious Diseases That Threaten the Blood Supply," *Seminars in Hematology*, Vol. 44, No. 1, 2007, pp. 32–41. As of October 18, 2016:
http://www.sciencedirect.com/science/article/pii/S0037196306002381

America's Blood Centers, "Stoplight Report," undated-a. As of October 18, 2016:
http://www.americasblood.org/stoplight.aspx

———, "Types of Blood Donations," undated-b. As of October 18, 2016:
http://www.americasblood.org/donate-blood/types-of-blood-donations.aspx

———, "America's Blood Centers Opposes Healthcare Reform Legislation That Imposes Fee or Tax on Medical Devices Sold to Blood Centers," Washington, D.C.: America's Blood Centers, 2009. As of May 5, 2016:
http://www.americasblood.org/media/27979/stmnt_091203_medicaldevicefee.pdf

American Association for Clinical Chemistry, "Transfusion Medicine," December 3, 2015. As of December 9, 2015:
https://labtestsonline.org/lab/bloodbank/start/6/

American Association of Blood Banks, "Disaster Response," undated-a. As of October 18, 2016:
http://www.aabb.org/programs/disasterresponse/Pages/default.aspx

———, "Donor Hemovigilance," undated-b. As of October 18, 2016:
http://www.aabb.org/research/hemovigilance/Pages/donor-hemovigilance.aspx

———, "Response to to Comments Received to the 30th Edition of Standards for Blood Banks and Transfusion Services," undated-c. As of October 18, 2016:
https://www.aabb.org/sa/standards/Documents/
Response-to-Comments-Standards-for-Blood-Banks-and-Transfusion-Services-30th-edition.pdf

———, *AABB Billing Guide for Transfusion and Cellular Therapy Services*, 2007. As of October 18, 2016:
http://www.aabb.org/advocacy/reimbursementinitiatives/Documents/reimbguidev071017.pdf

———, *Disaster Operations Handbook*, Bethesda, Md., October 2008. As of October 18, 2016:
http://www.aabb.org/programs/disasterresponse/documents/disastophndbkv2.pdf

———, *Interorganizational Task Force on Pandemic Influenza and The Blood Supply, Pandemic Influenza Planning*, Version 2.0, Bethesda, Md., October 2009. As of October 18, 2016:
http://www.aabb.org/programs/disasterresponse/documents/piplanning.pdf

American Red Cross, home page, undated-a. As of November 3, 2015:
http://www.redcrossblood.org/

———, "Significant Dates In Red Cross History," undated-b. As of October 18, 2016:
http://www.redcross.org/about-us/history/significant-dates-in-history

———, "Types of Donations," undated-c. As of November 4, 2015:
http://www.redcrossblood.org/donating-blood/types-donations

———, "Types of Emergencies," undated-d. As of October 18, 2016:
http://www.redcross.org/get-help/prepare-for-emergencies/types-of-emergencies

———, "Sandy Forces Cancellation of About 300 Blood Drives," October 30, 2012. As of October 18, 2016:
http://www.redcross.org/news/article/Sandy-Forces-Cancellation-of-About-300-Blood-Drives

American Society for Clinical Pathology, *The Medical Laboratory Personnel Shortage*, policy statement, April 2004. As of October 18, 2016:
https://www.ascp.org/content/docs/default-source/pdf/57723a0c-bd18-473c-be76-d66b52ae5594.pdf

Armed Services Blood Program, *We Are The Armed Services Blood Program*, Falls Church, Va., November 23, 2013. As of December 16, 2015:
http://www.militaryblood.dod.mil/articlearchive/presskit_11_25_13.pdf

———, "ASBP Components," 2015a. As of December 16, 2015:
http://www.militaryblood.dod.mil/About/components.aspx

———, *ASBP Educational Campaign Factsheet*, Falls Church, Va., 2015b. As of November 18, 2015:
http://www.militaryblood.dod.mil/press/Documents/Print_Factssheet.pdf

———, "Blood Distribution Chart Text Version," 2015c. As of December 16, 2015:
http://www.militaryblood.dod.mil/About/distrib_chart_text.aspx

———, "Can I Donate?" 2015d. As of December 16, 2015:
http://www.militaryblood.dod.mil/Donors/can_i_donate.aspx

———, "Frequently Asked Questions," 2015e. As of December 10, 2015:
http://www.militaryblood.dod.mil/Donors/donor_faq.aspx

———, home page, 2015f. As of November 2, 2015:
http://www.militaryblood.dod.mil/default.aspx

An, Ming-Wen, Nicholas G. Reich, Stephen O. Crawford, Ron Brookmeyer, Thomas A. Louis, and Kenrad E. Nelson, "A Stochastic Simulator of a Blood Product Donation Environment with Demand Spikes and Supply Shocks," *PloS One*, Vol. 6, No. 7, 2011, p. e21752. As of October 18, 2016:
http://journals.plos.org/plosone/article?id=10.1371%2Fjournal.pone.0021752

ASBP—*See* Armed Services Blood Program.

AuBuchon, J. P., K. Puca, S. Saxena, I. Shulman, and J. Waters, *Getting Started in Patient Blood Management*, Bethesda, Md.: American Association of Blood Banks, 2011.

AuBuchon, J. P., M. Fung, B. Whitaker, and J. Malasky, "AABB Validation Study of the CDC's National Healthcare Safety Network Hemovigilance Module Adverse Events Definitions Protocol," *Transfusion*, Vol. 54, No. 8, 2014, pp. 2077–2083.

Australian Ministry of Health, National Blood Agreement Between the Commonwealth of Australia and the States and Territories, 2003. As of October 18, 2016:
http://www.cec.health.nsw.gov.au/__data/assets/pdf_file/0008/258074/
national_blood_agreement-australia.pdf

Australian Red Cross Blood Service, "History," undated. As of October 18, 2016:
http://www.donateblood.com.au/about/history

Australian Red Cross, "Residual Risk Estimates for Transfusion-Transmissible Infections," February 2016. As of October 18, 2016:
http://www.transfusion.com.au/adverse_events/risks/estimates

Autor, Deborah, "Securing the Pharmaceutical Supply Chain," hearing before the Committee on Health, Education, Labor and Pensions, U.S. Senate, Washington, D.C.: Food and Drug Administration, September 14, 2011. As of October 18, 2016:
http://www.fda.gov/NewsEvents/Testimony/ucm271073.htm

Banta, H. David, "Examples of per-Case and DRG Payment Systems," in *Diagnosis Related Groups (DRGs) and the Medicare Program: Implications for Medical Technology, Appendix C*, 1983. As of October 26, 2016:
https://www.princeton.edu/~ota/disk3/1983/8306/830611.PDF

Bhatnagar, Nidhi M., and Maitry D Gajjar, "Hemovigilance: Need of the Hour," *Biennial Journal of GAPM*, undated. As of October 18, 2016:
http://www.palmonline.org/node/172

Biologics Direct, "Nation's Blood Distribution Undergoes Major Changes," Alex Garcia and Charles Rouault, March 16, 2015. As of May 5, 2016:
http://www.prweb.com/releases/2015/03/prweb12578852.htm

Bloodbuy, "Bloodbuy for Hospitals," undated. As of May 5, 2016:
http://www.Bloodbuy.com/for-hospitals/

"Blood Centers Announce Merger Intent," *Thomasville Times-Enterprise*, July 25, 2014.

Blood Centers of America, home page, 2015. As of October 24, 2016:
http://bca.coop/

"Blood Donation Lines Grow in Orlando After Shooting," ABC 7 News, June 12, 2016. As of October 18, 2016:
http://abc7.com/news/blood-donation-lines-grow-in-orlando-after-shooting/1382223/

BloodSource Inc., "BloodSource and Shasta Blood Center to Combine Redding Operations," Mather, Calif., December 3, 2015. As of May 5, 2016:
https://www.bloodsource.org/News/News-Releases/
Media-Release-BloodSource-and-Shasta-Blood-Center

Blood Systems Research Institute, *BSRI Program Review*, Blood Systems Inc., 2011. As of October 18, 2016:
http://www.bsrisf.org/pdfs/bsri_program_review_2011.pdf

"Blood Transfusion Sale Set to Give Novartis a £1bn Shot in the Arm," City A.M. Reporter, November 12, 2013.

Boris, Elizabeth T., and C. Eugene Steuerle, eds., "After Katrina: Public Expectation and Charities' Response," The Urban Institute, May 2006. As of October 18, 2016:
http://www.urban.org/sites/default/files/alfresco/publication-pdfs/311331-After-Katrina-Public-Expectation-and-Charities-Response.PDF

Brinkmann, Paul, "How Blood Banks Handled Pulse Shooting, 28,000 Donors," *Orlando Sentinel*, July 1, 2016. As of October 18, 2016:
http://www.orlandosentinel.com/news/pulse-orlando-nightclub-shooting/os-oneblood-ceo-pulse-20160629-story.html

Bureau of Labor Statistics, "Hospital Producer Price Index," 2016. As of October 18, 2016:
http://download.bls.gov/pub/time.series/pc/pc.data.50.Hospitals

Caiola, Sammy, "Blood Banks Face 'Unprecedented' Shortage Due in Part to Zika Restrictions," *Sacramento Bee*, July 5, 2016. As of October 18, 2016:
http://www.sacbee.com/news/local/health-and-medicine/article87883977.html

"Canada's Tainted Blood Scandal: A Timeline," CBC News, October 1, 2007. As of October 18, 2016:
http://www.cbc.ca/news2/background/taintedblood/bloodscandal_timeline.html

Canadian Blood Services, *A Report to Canadians 2007/2008: Transforming Canada's Blood System*, Ottawa, Canada: Office of Strategy Management, 2008. As of October 18, 2016:
https://www.blood.ca/sites/default/files/07-08-CBS-Annual-Report-en.pdf

Canadian Red Cross, "A Time of Change: 1990–1999," undated. As of October 18, 2016:
http://www.redcross.ca/about-us/about-the-canadian-red-cross/historical-highlights/a-time-of-change--1990-1999

CAP Today, "Haemonetics Software Solutions, SafeTrace Tx Blood Bank Information Systems," October 2015. As of October 24, 2016:
http://www.captodayonline.com/productguides/software-systems/blood-bank-information-systems-october-2015/haemonetics-software-solutions-safetrace-tx-blood-bank-october-2015.html

Castagna, Jr., Peter J., and Pascal George, "Lehigh Valley and Central New Jersey Blood Centers Announce Intent to Merge Operations," Bethlehem, Pa.: Miller-Keystone Blood Center, November 5, 2014. As of May 5, 2016:
http://www.giveapint.org/wp-content/uploads/2014/01/MKBC-CJBC_Merger_11.5.2014.pdf

CDC—*See* Centers for Disease Control and Prevention.

CDC, NHSN—*See* Centers for Disease Control and Prevention, National Healthcare Safety Network.

Centers for Disease Control and Prevention, *The National Healthcare Safety Network (NHSN) Manual: Biovigilance Component Hemovigilance Module Surveillance Protocol, Version 2.2*, Atlanta, Ga.: Division of Healthcare Quality Promotion, National Center for Emerging and Zoonotic Infectious Diseases, June 2006. As of October 18, 2016:
http://www.cdc.gov/nhsn/PDFs/Biovigilance/BV-HV-protocol-current.pdf

———, *Biovigilance Component Hemovigilance Module Adverse Reaction and Denominator Reporting*, 2013. As of October 26, 2016:
http://www.cdc.gov/nhsn/pdfs/training/biovig/adverse-reactions_october2013.pdf

Centers for Disease Control and Prevention, National Healthcare Safety Network, "Frequently Asked Questions About Hemovigilance Module," last updated February 2016. As of October 26, 2016:
http://www.cdc.gov/nhsn/faqs/biovig/faq_hemovigilance.html#q4

————, "Blood Safety Surveillance," last updated September 2016. As of October 18, 2016: http://www.cdc.gov/nhsn/acute-care-hospital/bio-hemo/

Centers for Medicare and Medicaid Services, "CMS-1632-F and IFC, CMS-1632-CN2 and Changes Due to the Consolidated Appropriations Act of 2016: Final Rule, Correction Notice and the Consolidated Appropriations Act of 2016," Baltimore, Md., 2016a.

————, "Hospital Outpatient Prospective Payment—Final Rule with Comment Period and Final CY2016 Payment Rates," Baltimore, Md., 2016b. As of October 25, 2016: https://www.cms.gov/Medicare/Medicare-Fee-for-Service-Payment/HospitalOutpatientPPS/ Hospital-Outpatient-Regulations-and-Notices-Items/CMS-1633-FC.html

Chung, K.-W., S. V. Basavaraju, Y. Mu, K. L. van Santen, K. A. Haass, R. Henry, J. Berger, and M. J. Kuehnert, "Declining Blood Collection and Utilization in the United States, *Transfusion*, Vol. 56, No. 9, May 12, 2016, pp. 2184–2192.

Clarke, Toni, "Zika-Hit Puerto Rico Prepares to Import All of Its Blood Supplies," Reuters, February 19, 2016. As of October 18, 2016: http://www.reuters.com/article/us-health-zika-blood-insight-idUSKCN0VS0FI

Clyde, A., L. Bockstedt, J. Farkas, and C. Jackson, "Experience with Medicare's New Technology Add-on Payment Program," *Health Affairs*, Vol. 27, No. 6, 2008.

Como, J.J., R. P. Dutton, T. M. Scalea, B. B. Edelman, J. R. Hess, "Blood Transfusion Rates in the Care of Acute Trauma," *Transfusion,* Vol. 44, No. 6, 2004, pp. 809–813.

Cost of Blood Consensus Conference, "The Cost of Blood: Multidisciplinary Consensus Conference for a Standard Methodology," *Transfusion Medicine Reviews,* Vol. 19, No. 1, January 2005, pp. 66–78. As of October 17, 2016: http://ac.els-cdn.com/S0887796304000562/1-s2.0-S0887796304000562-main.pdf?_ tid=385e9048-871d-11e5-aaba-00000aab0f02&acdnat=1447099707_7ae616df63e25ed2f3b174a c1f900442

Crary, David, "After Superstorm Sandy Surge, Donations to Red Cross Drop," *Athens Banner-Herald*, October 29, 2015. As of October 18, 2016: http://onlineathens.com/national-news/2015-10-29/ after-superstorm-sandy-surge-donations-red-cross-drop

Custer, Brian, Artina Chinn, Nora V. Hirschler, Michael P. Busch, and Edward L. Murphy, "The Consequences of Temporary Deferral on Future Whole Blood Donation," *Transfusion*, Vol. 47, No. 8, 2007, pp. 1514–1523.

Cutler, David M., and Fiona Scott Morton, "Hospitals, Market Share, and Consolidation," *JAMA,* Vol. 310, No. 18, 2013, pp. 1964–1970.

Dent, Charles W., U.S. Representative of Pennsylvania, Consolidated Appropriations Act 2016, code edition dated January 5, 2015. As of May 5, 2016: https://www.congress.gov/bill/114th-congress/house-bill/2029/ text#toc-H06D7A0621C1E4307B3153017167BB3A8

Ditomasso, Julie, Yang Liu, and Nancy M. Heddle, "The Canadian Transfusion Surveillance System: What Is It and How Can the Data Be Used?" *Transfusion and Apheresis Science*, Vol. 46, No. 3, 2012, pp. 329–335.

DoD—*See* U.S. Department of Defense.

Dodd, Roger Y., "Emerging Pathogens and Their Implications for the Blood Supply and Transfusion Transmitted Infections," *British Journal of Haematology*, Vol. 159, No. 2, 2007, pp. 135–142.

Dodd, Roger Y., and Louis M. Katz, "Qui Custodiet Ipsos Custodes?" *Transfusion*, Vol. 55, No. 4, 2015, pp. 693–695. As of October 18, 2016: http://onlinelibrary.wiley.com/doi/10.1111/trf.13023/abstract

Duchesne, Juan C., John P. Hunt, Georgia Wahl, Alan B. Marr, Yi-Zarn Wang, Sharon E. Weintraub, Mary Jo Wright, and Norman E. McSwain Jr., "Review of Current Blood Transfusions Strategies in a Mature Level I Trauma Center: Were We Wrong for the Last 60 Years?" *Journal of Trauma and Acute Care Surgery*, Vol. 65, No. 2, 2008, pp. 272–278.

Engelbrecht, Sunelle, Erica Wood, and Merole F. Cole-Sinclair, "Clinical Transfusion Practice Update: Haemovigilance, Complications, Patient Blood Management and National Standards," *Medical Journal of Australia*, Vol. 199, No. 6, 2013, pp. 397–401. As of October 26, 2016: https://www.mja.com.au/journal/2013/199/6/clinical-transfusion-practice-update-haemovigilance-complications-patient-blood

Erickson, Michelle L., Melanie H. Champion, Roger Klein, Rebecca L. Ross, Zena M. Neal, and Edward L. Snyder, "Management of Blood Shortages in a Tertiary Care Academic Medical Center: The Yale–New Haven Hospital Frozen Blood Reserve," *Transfusion*, Vol. 48, No. 10, 2008, pp. 2252–2263. As of October 18, 2016: http://dx.doi.org/10.1111/j.1537-2995.2008.01816.x

European Medicines Agency, "Work Plan for the CHMP Blood Products Working Party (BPWP) for 2016," London, UK, February 2016. As of October 18, 2016: http://www.ema.europa.eu/docs/en_GB/document_library/Work_programme/2010/02/WC500073390.pdf

Farris, Meg, "Critical Shortage: Blood Center Down to 1-Day Supply," WWLTV, June 10, 2016. As of October 18, 2016: http://www.wwltv.com/news/health/critical-shortage-blood-center-down-to-1-day-supply/239177486

FDA—*See* U.S. Food and Drug Administration.

Federal Emergency Management Agency, "Emergency Support Function No. 8—Public Health and Medical Services Annex," January 2008. As of October 18, 2016: https://www.fema.gov/media-library-data/20130726-1825-25045-8027/emergency_support_function_8_public_health___medical_services_annex_2008.pdf

Ferguson, Eamon, and Peter A. Bibby, "Predicting Future Blood Donor Returns: Past Behavior, Intentions, and Observer Effects," *Health Psychology*, Vol. 21, No. 5, 2002, p. 513.

Ferguson, Eamonn, Christopher R. France, Charles Abraham, Blaine Ditto, and Paschal Sheeran, "Improving Blood Donor Recruitment and Retention: Integrating Theoretical Advances from Social and Behavioral Science Research Agendas," *Transfusion*, Vol. 47, No. 11, 2007, pp. 1999–2010.

FindLaw, "International Product Liability Laws," undated. As of October 18, 2016: http://corporate.findlaw.com/litigation-disputes/international-product-liability-laws.html

Firger, Jessica, "FDA Approves First Zika Diagnostic Test for Commercial Use," *Newsweek*, February 26, 2016. As of October 18, 2016: http://www.newsweek.com/zika-virus-diagnosis-antibody-test-fda-approved-431053

Flood, Philip, Peter Wills, Peter Lawler, Graeme Ryan, and Kevin Rickard, "Review of Australia's Plasma Fractionation Arrangements," Australian Government Department of Health, 2006. As of October 10, 2016: http://www.health.gov.au/plasmafractionationreview

Fontaine, Magali J., Y. T. Chung, F. Erhun, and L.T. Goodnough, "Age of Blood as a Limitation for Transfusion: Potential Impact on Blood Inventory and Availability," *Transfusion*, Vol. 50, No. 10, 2010, pp. 2233–2239.

France, Christopher R., Janis L. France, Marios Roussos, and Blaine Ditto, "Mild Reactions to Blood Donation Predict a Decreased Likelihood of Donor Return," *Transfusion and Apheresis Science*, Vol. 30, No. 1, 2004, pp. 17–22.

Fung, Mark, Brenda Grossman, Christopher Hillyer, and Connie Westhoff, *AABB Technical Manual*, 18th ed., 2014.

Garcia, Edna, Asma M. Ali, Ryan M. Soles, and D. Grace Lewis, "The American Society for Clinical Pathology's 2014 Vacancy Survey of Medical Laboratories in the United States," *American Journal of Clinical Pathology*, Vol. 144, No. 3, September 1, 2015, pp. 432–443.

Glasgow, S. M., S. Allard, H. Doughty, P. Spreadborough, and E. Watkins, "Blood and Bombs: The Demand and Use of Blood Following the London Bombings of 7 July 2005–A Retrospective Review," *Transfusion Medicine*, Vol. 22, No. 4, 2012, pp. 244–250.

Goodman, C., S. Chan, P. Collins, R. Haught, and Y. J. Chen, "Ensuring Blood Safety and Availability in the U.S.: Technological Advances, Costs, and Challenges to Payment—Final Report," *Transfusion*, Vol. 43, No. 8, Supplement, August 2003, pp. 3s–46s.

Goodman, D. C., A. Esty, E. S. Fisher, and C. H. Chang, "A Report of the Dartmouth Atlas Project," Hanover, N.H.: Dartmouth Institute for Health Policy and Clinical Practice, 2010.

Goodman, D. C., E. S. Fisher, C. H. Chang, S. R. Raymond, and K. K. Bronner, "After Hospitalization: A Dartmouth Atlas Report on Post-Acute Care for Medicare Beneficiaries," Hanover, N.H.: Dartmouth Institute for Health Policy and Clinical Practice, Vol. 28, 2011.

Goodnough, L. T., "Blood Management: Transfusion Medicine Comes of Age," *Lancet,* Vol. 381, No. 9880, May 25, 2013, pp. 1791–1792.

Goodnough, L. T., J. H. Levy, and M. F. Murphy, "Concepts of Blood Transfusion in Adults," *Lancet,* Vol. 381, No. 9880, May 25, 2013, pp. 1845–1854.

Grazzini, Giuliano, and Simonetta Pupella, "Setting Up and Implementation of the National Hemovigilance System in Italy," in Rene R. P. de Vries and Jean-Claude Faber, eds., *Hemovigilance: An Effective Tool for Improving Transfusion Safety*, 2012, pp. 204–208. As of October 18, 2016: https://books.google.com/books?id=KHbDaPnVdXoC&lpg=PT301&ots=4j0jLucCYc&dq=Cen tro%20Nazionale%20Sangue%20national%20center%20blood&hl=cs&pg=PT301#v=onepage&q= Centro%20Nazionale%20Sangue%20national%20center%20blood&f=false

Green, David, "Blood Systems' Perspective on State of the Current Blood System," Washington, D.C.: Blood Systems Inc., November 9, 2015.

Harvey, Alexis, Sridhar V. Basavaraju, Koo-Whang Chung, and Matthew J. Kuehnert, "Transfusion-Related Adverse Reactions Reported to the National Healthcare Safety Network Hemovigilance Module, United States, 2010 to 2012," *Transfusion*, Vol. 55, No. 4, 2015, pp. 709–718.

Health Resources and Services Administration, *The Clinical Laboratory Workforce: The Changing Picture of Supply, Demand, Education and Practice*, Washington, D.C.: U.S. Department of Health and Human Services, July 2005. As of October 18, 2016: http://bhpr.hrsa.gov/healthworkforce/reports/clinicallab.pdf

Health Resources and Services Administration, "FY 2017 Budget Review," last reviewed March 2016. As of October 18, 2016: http://www.hrsa.gov/about/budget/hrsabudgetoverview-2017.pdf

Heflin, Theresa, and Christie Newman, "Trends, Directions in Blood Banking," King of Prussia, Pa.: Advance Healthcare Network, December 1, 2002. As of May 5, 2016: http://laboratory-manager.advanceweb.com/Article/Trends-Directions-in-Blood-Banking-1.aspx

Héma-Québec, "Research and Development at Héma-Québec: An Overview," 2014. As of October 18, 2016:
http://www.hema-quebec.qc.ca/recherche-developpement/index.en.html

Hernandez, J., S. Machacz, and J. Robinson, "U.S. Hospital Payment Adjustments for Innovative Technology Lag Behind Those in Germany, France, and Japan," *Health Affairs*, Vol. 34, No. 2, 2015.

HHS—*See* U.S. Department of Health and Human Services.

Hiers, Fred, "OneBlood Seeks Partner, a Sign of the Times," *Ocala Star-Banner*, 2014.

Hologic, Inc., "FDA Expands Emergency Use Authorization for Hologic's Aptima Zika Virus Assay to Include Use with Urine Samples," press release, September 8, 2016. As of October 25, 2016:
http://investors.hologic.com/2016-09-08-FDA-Expands-Emergency-Use-Authorization-for-Hologics-Aptima-Zika-Virus-Assay-to-Include-Use-with-Urine-Samples

Homeland Security Council, "National Planning Scenarios: Executive Summaries," Version 20.2, 2006a. As of October 18, 2016:
http://cees.tamiu.edu/covertheborder/TOOLS/NationalPlanningSen.pdf

Homeland Security Council, *National Strategy for Pandemic Influenza: Implementation Plan*, Washington, D.C.: U.S. Department of Homeland Security, 2006b. As of October 18, 2016:
http://www.flu.gov/planning-preparedness/federal/pandemic-influenza-implementation.pdf

Hrouda, Chris, presentation to the U.S. Department of Health and Human Services Advisory Committee on Blood and Tissue Safety and Availability, Washington, D.C., 2015.

India Pharma News, "Transparency Market Research: Global RFID Blood Monitoring Systems Market Is Expected to Reach USD 40.9 Million in 2012," Contify.com, January 11, 2014.

International Medical Device Regulators Forum, home page, undated-a. As of October 18, 2016:
http://www.imdrf.org/

International Medical Device Regulators Forum, "About IMDRF," undated-b. As of October 18, 2016:
http://www.imdrf.org/about/about.asp

Internal Revenue Service, "Medical Device Excise Tax: Tax Law Change to the Medical Device Excise Tax," January 11, 2016. As of May 5, 2016:
https://www.irs.gov/uac/Newsroom/Medical-Device-Excise-Tax

International Society for Pharmacoeconomics, "Structure and Focus of the German Red Cross Blood Transfusion Service Baden-Württemberg-Hessia And Its Affiliates," 2010. As of October 18, 2016:
https://www.blutspende.de/en/_files/structure.pdf

International Society for Pharmacoeconomics, "Italy—Medical Devices and Diagnostics," 2012. As of October 18, 2016:
https://www.ispor.org/HTARoadMaps/Italy/Italy_MDD.asp

Japanese Red Cross Society, *Blood Services 2015*, Minato-Ku, Tokyo: Blood Service Headquarters, 2015. As of October 18, 2016:
http://www.jrc.or.jp/english/pdf/Blood_Services_2015_web.pdf

Jones, Lucile M., Richard Bernknopf, Dale Cox, James Goltz, Kenneth Hudnut, Dennis Mileti, Suzanne Perry, Daniel Ponti, Keith Porter, and Michael Reichle, "The Shakeout Scenario," *U.S. Geological Survey Open-File Report*, California Geological Survey, Vol. 1150, No. 25, 2008. As of October 18, 2016:
http://pubs.usgs.gov/of/2008/1150/of2008-1150small.pdf

Kamel, Hany, Marjorie Bravo, Brian Custer, and Peter Tomasulo, *Donor Vigilance: Five-Year Journey of Continuous Process Improvement*, Blood Systems, 2011. As of October 18, 2016:
http://www.ihn-org.com/wp-content/uploads/2011/02/14h45-BSI_Vigilance__HKamel.pdf

Kamp, Christel, Margarethe Heiden, Olaf Henseler, and Rainer Seitz, "Management of Blood Supplies During an Influenza Pandemic," *Transfusion*, Vol. 50, No. 1, 2010, pp. 231–239.

Kamper-Jorgensen, M., H. Hjalgrim, G. Edgren, K. Titlestad, H. Ullum, A. Shanwell, M. Reilly, M. Melbye, O. Nyren, and K. Rostgaard, "Expensive Blood Safety Initiatives May Offer Less Benefit Than We Think," *Transfusion,* Vol. 50, No. 1, January 2010, pp. 240–242. As of October 25, 2016:
http://onlinelibrary.wiley.com/doi/10.1111/j.1537-2995.2009.02374.x/abstract

Kato, Hidefumi, Motoaki Uruma, Yoshiki Okuyama, Hiroshi Fujita, Makoto Handa, Yoshiaki Tomiyama, Shigetaka Shimodaira, Yoshiyuki Kurata, and Shigeru Takamoto, "Incidence of Transfusion-Related Adverse Reactions per Patient Reflects the Potential Risk of Transfusion Therapy in Japan," *American Journal of Clinical Pathology*, Vol. 140, No. 2, 2013, pp. 219–224.

Kaufman, Kenneth, "Fast and Furious Blood Industry Decline Sends a Message to the Healthcare Industry," *Health Finance Manage*, Vol. 68, No. 12, December 2014, p. 104. As of October 18, 2016:
https://support.kaufmanhall.com/hlc/Content/Documents/
Fast%20and%20Furious%20Blood%20Industry.pdf

Kaufman, Kenneth, "Blood Banks Unite to Better Serve Coachella Valley," *Desert Sun*, May 17, 2012.

Keller-Stanislawski, B., A. Lohmann, S. Günay, M. Heiden, and M. B. Funk, "The German Haemovigilance System–Reports of Serious Adverse Transfusion Reactions Between 1997 and 2007," *Transfusion Medicine*, Vol. 19, No. 6, 2009, pp. 340–349.

Khan, Anas, "Level of Willingness to Report to Work During a Pandemic Among the Emergency Department Health Care Professionals," *Asian Journal of Medical Sciences,* Vol. 5, No. 3, 2014, pp. 58–62.

Kidder, Kristen, "Donor Surge: The Challenge of Managing Blood Donations During Disaster," Federal Emergency Management Agency, May 13, 2010.

Klein, H. G., W. A. Flegel, and C. Natanson, "Red Blood Cell Transfusion: Precision vs Imprecision Medicine," *JAMA,* Vol. 314, No. 15, October 20, 2015, pp. 1557–1558.

Knowledge Based Systems Inc., "Blood Availability & Safety Information System (BASIS)," undated. As of October 18, 2016:
http://www.kbsi.com/kbsi/index.php?option=com_content&view=article&id=259&Itemid=2967

Kuruppu, Kumudu K. S., "Management of Blood System in Disasters," *Biologicals*, Vol. 38, No. 1, 2010, pp. 87–90.

Kwan, Joshua L., "Blood Banks Desperate Runaway Costs: Need Outpaces Donations," *San Jose Mercury News*, December 6, 1999.

Lemmens, K. P. H., C. Abraham, T. Hoekstra, R.A.C. Ruiter, W. L. A. M. De Kort, J. Brug, and H. P. Schaalma, "Why Don't Young People Volunteer to Give Blood? An Investigation of the Correlates of Donation Intentions Among Young Nondonors," *Transfusion*, Vol. 45, No. 6, 2005, pp. 945–955.

Litman, Todd, "Lessons from Katrina and Rita: What Major Disasters Can Teach Transportation Planners," *Journal of Transportation Engineering*, Vol. 132, No. 1, 2006, pp. 11–18. As of October 18, 2016:
http://www.vtpi.org/katrina.pdf

Lohmann, Annette Herr, Jochen Halbauer, Frau Cornelia Witzenhausen, Frau Klaudia Wesp, Herr Olaf Henseler, and Brigitte Keller-Stanislawski, *Paul Ehrlich Institut (PEI) Federal Institute for Vaccines and Biomedicines, Haemovigilance Report of the Paul Ehrlich Institut 2010*, Assessment of the Reports of Serious Adverse Transfusion Reactions Pursuant to Section 63c, AMG, Arzneimittelgesetz, German Medicinal Products Act, 2010.

Macpherson, J., C. B. Mahoney, L. Katz, J. Haarmann, and C. Bianco, "Contribution of Blood to Hospital Revenue in the United States," *Transfusion,* Vol. 47, No. 2, 2007, pp. 114S–116S. As of October 24, 2016:
http://onlinelibrary.wiley.com/doi/10.1111/j.1537-2995.2007.01364.x/abstract

MacQueen, K., E. McLellan, L. Kay, and B. Milstein, "Code Book Development for Team-Based Qualitative Analysis," *CAM Journal*, Vol. 10, 1988, pp. 31–36.

Marks, P. W., J. S. Epstein, and L. Borio, "Maintaining a Safe Blood Supply in an Era of Emerging Pathogens," *Journal of Infectious Diseases*, March 8, 2016.

Massey, Gemma, "Marketing Environments: The European Airline Industry," Marked By Teachers, 2015. As of May 5, 2016:
http://www.markedbyteachers.com/university-degree/business-and-administrative-studies/european-airline.html

McCue, M. J., and P. Nayar, "Hospital Billing for Blood Processing and Transfusion for Inpatient Stays," *Transfusion,* Vol. 49, No. 7, Part 2, July 2009, pp. 1517–1519.

McCullough, J., J. M. McCullough, and W. J. Riley, "Evolution of the Nation's Blood Supply System," *Transfusion*, Vol. 56, No. 6, April 4, 2016, pp. 1459–1461.

Medicines and Healthcare Products Regulatory Agency (MHRA) and Serious Hazards of Transfusion (SHOT), *Annual SHOT Report*, Serious Hazards of Transfusion, 2014. As of October 18, 2016:
http://www.shotuk.org/wp-content/uploads/a.pdf

Mehra, T., B. Seifert, S. Bravo-Reiter, G. Wanner, P. Dutkowski, T. Holubec, R. M. Moos, J. Volbracht, M. G. Manz, and D. R. Spahn, "Implementation of a Patient Blood Management Monitoring and Feedback Program Significantly Reduces Transfusions and Costs," *Transfusion*, Vol. 55, No. 12, 2015, pp. 2807–2815.

Miles, M. B., and A. M. Huberman, *Qualitative Data Analysis: An Expanded Sourcebook*, Thousand Oaks, Calif.: Sage Publications, 1994.

Morris, Chris, and Shawn Berry, "Nebraska Blood Service a Model for Success," *Telegraph-Journal (New Brunswick)*, November 26, 2011.

Murphy, M. F., "The Choosing Wisely Campaign to Reduce Harmful Medical Overuse: Its Close Association with Patient Blood Management Initiatives," *Transfusion Medicine*, Vol. 25, No. 5, October 16, 2015, pp. 287–292.

Murphy, M. F., E. Fraser, D. Miles, S. Noel, J. Staves, B. Cripps, and J. Kay, "How Do We Monitor Hospital Transfusion Practice Using an End-to-End Electronic Transfusion Management System?" *Transfusion*, Vol. 52, No. 12, 2012, pp. 2502–2512.

Musso, Didier, Susan L. Stramer, and Michael P. Busch, "Zika Virus: A New Challenge for Blood Transfusion," *Lancet*, Vol. 387, No. 10032, May 2016, pp. 1993–1994. As of October 18, 2016:
http://www.thelancet.com/journals/lancet/article/PIIS0140-6736(16)30428-7/fulltext?rss%3Dyes

Nahmias, Laura, "Poor Communication Fueled Post-Sandy Gas Shortage," *Wall Street Journal*, March 20, 2013. As of October 18, 2016:
http://www.wsj.com/articles/SB10001424127887324323904578368450399698818

Nakano, Rina, "Blood Banks Cite Zika Virus as Reason for Shortage," Fox 40 Sacramento, July 8, 2016:
http://fox40.com/2016/07/08/blood-banks-cite-zika-virus-as-reason-for-shortage/

National Association of Social Workers, "Blood Banks Serving Polk County to Merge," *The Ledger*, 2015. As of May 5, 2016:
http://cqrcengage.com/socialworkersnc/app/
document/8775930;jsessionid=JlO2lisLdHI0YsXtdeCxN-hC.undefined

National Blood Authority, "Overview: Ensuring Supply," undated. As of October 18, 2016:
https://www.blood.gov.au/ensuring-supply

———, *Australian Haemovigilance Minimum Data Set*, Canberra, Australia, August 2015a. As of October 24, 2016:
https://www.blood.gov.au/system/files/aust-haemovigilance-min-data-set.pdf

———, *National Blood Authority, Australia, Annual Report 2014–15*, Canberra, Australia, October 7, 2015b. As of October 18, 2016:
https://www.blood.gov.au/sites/default/files/nba-annualreport-2014-15-as-at-20151013sm_1.pdf

National Blood Authority Haemovigilance Advisory Committee, *Australian Haemovigilance Report, Data for 2011–12 and 2012–13*, National Blood Authority, 2013. As of October 18, 2016:
https://www.blood.gov.au/pubs/2015-haemovigilance/index/australian-haemovigilance-report.html

NBA—*See* National Blood Authority.

National Heart, Lung, and Blood Institute, "NHLBI Blood Diseases and Resources Program: Obligations by Funding Mechanism, Fiscal Year 2012," 2012. As of October 10, 2016:
https://www.nhlbi.nih.gov/about/documents/factbook/2012/chapter7#blooddisrecprog

National Health Service, "History," undated. As of October 18, 2016:
http://www.nhsbt.nhs.uk/who-we-are/history

Neale, Rick, "Blood Donations Skyrocket in Florida After Orlando Massacre," *Florida Today*, KHOU, 06/30/2016, 2016. As of October 18, 2016:
http://www.khou.com/news/blood-donations-skyrocket-in-florida-after-orlando-massacre/260930801

Negin, Steve, "The Changing Landscape of Blood Banking," *Advance Healthcare Network*, Vol. 24, No. 4, March 26, 2015, p. 28. As of May 3, 2016:
http://laboratory-manager.advanceweb.com/Archives/Article-Archives/The-Changing-Landscape-of-Blood-Banking.aspx

"Nepal Quake: Airport Customs Holding up Aid Relief—UN," BBC, May 3, 2015. As of October 18, 2016:
http://www.bbc.com/news/world-asia-32564891

Newman, Bruce, "Blood Donor Suitability and Allogeneic Whole Blood Donation," *Transfusion Medicine Reviews,* Vol. 15, No. 3, 2001, pp. 234–244.

"New York Blood Center in Short Supply, in Need of Donations," *CBS New York*, June 15, 2016. As of October 18, 2016:
http://newyork.cbslocal.com/2016/06/15/new-york-blood-center-donations/;

Nguyen, Dorothy D., Deborah A. DeVita, Nora V. Hirschler, and Edward L. Murphy, "Blood Donor Satisfaction and Intention of Future Donation," *Transfusion*, Vol. 48, No. 4, 2008, pp. 742–748.

NHLBI—*See* National Heart, Lung, and Blood Institute.

Nielsen, A. E., and N. D. Nielsen, "Assessing Productive Efficiency and Operating Scale of Community Blood Centers," *Transfusion*, Vol. 56, No. 6, June 2016.

Nightingale, Stephen, Virginia Wanamaker, Barbara Silverman, Paul McCurdy, Lawrence McMurtry, Philip Quarles, S. Gerald Sandler, Darrell Triulzi, Carolyn Whitsett, Christopher Hillyer, Leo McCarthy, Dennis Goldfinger, and David Satcher, "Use of Sentinel Sites for Daily Monitoring of the U.S. Blood Supply," *Transfusion*, Vol. 43, No. 3, pp. 364–372.

Nollet, Kenneth E., Hitoshi Ohto, Hiroyasu Yasuda, and Arifumi Hasegawa, "The Great East Japan Earthquake of March 11, 2011, from the Vantage Point of Blood Banking and Transfusion Medicine," *Transfusion Medicine Reviews*, Vol. 27, No. 1, 2013, pp. 29–35.

Office of the Assistant Secretary for Planning and Evaluation, "Health Insurance Coverage and the Affordable Care Act," ASPE Data Point, September 2015. As of October 10, 2016: https://aspe.hhs.gov/sites/default/files/pdf/111826/ACA%20health%20insurance%20coverage%20 brief%2009212015.pdf

Office of Parliamentary Counsel, *National Blood Authority Act 2003*, July 19, 2016. As of October 18, 2016: https://www.legislation.gov.au/Details/C2016C00846

Okazaki, Hitoshi, Naoko Goto, Shun-Ya Momose, Satoru Hino, and Kenji Tadokoro, "The Japanese Hemovigilance System," in R. R. P. De Vries and J.-C. Faber, eds., *Hemovigilance: An Effective Tool for Improving Transfusion Safety*, Oxford, UK: Wiley-Blackwell, 2012, pp. 159–167. As of October 18, 2016: http://dx.doi.org/10.1002/9781118338179.ch13

OneBlood and the Institute for Transfusion Medicine, "Blood Centers Announce Intent to Merge," LifeSource, July 25, 2014

Oravecz, John D., "Central Blood Bank Parent in Merger Talks with Florida System," *Trib Live*, July 28, 2014. As of May 5, 2016: http://triblive.com/business/headlines/6519430-74/blood-centers-covert#axzz3xtgYCjmX

Parkman, Paul D, "Control of Unsuitable Blood and Blood Components," Silver Spring, Md.: U.S. Food and Drug Administration, April 6, 1988. As of January 13, 2016: http://www.fda.gov/downloads/Biolog...toBloodEstablishments/UCM063008.pdf

Parmer, Tracy, "Coming Together to Save Lives," Armed Services Blood Program, May 22, 2015. As of December 14, 2015: http://www.militaryblood.dod.mil/viewcontent.aspx?con_id_pk=1879

Pera, Eric, "Local Blood Bank to Take Part in Nationwide Test; The Test Will Safeguard Against HIV, Hepatitis C.," *The Ledger*, April 1, 1999.

Pfuntner, Anne, Lauren Wier, and Carol Stocks, "Most Frequent Procedures Performed in U.S. Hospitals, 2011," Statistical Brief No. 165, Agency for Healthcare Research and Quality, October 2013. As of October 10, 2016: http://www.hcup-us.ahrq.gov/reports/statbriefs/sb165.pdf

Plapp, Fred V., "Future of Transfusion Medicine & Blood Banking," Heart of America Association of Blood Banks, 2013. As of May 5, 2016: http://www.haabb.org/images/11-_Fred_Plapp_-_Future_Transfusion_Med_BB.pdf

Plasma Protein Theraputics Association, home page, undated. As of November 4, 2015: http://www.donatingplasma.org/

Quaranta, J. F., F. Berthier, R. Courbil, F. Courtois, F. Chenais, C. Waller, M. F. Leconte des Floris, G. Andreu, O. Fontaine, C. Le Niger, M. Puntous, A. Mercadier, L. Nguyen, E. Pelissier, G. Gondrexon, and P. Staccini, "Qui sont les receveurs de produits sanguins labiles (PSL)? Une étude nationale multicentrique—un jour donné. Établissement de transfusion sanguine (ETS)— établissements de santé (ES) [Who are the recipients of labile blood products? [A Multicenter Nationwide Study—A 'Donation Day.' Blood Banks, Health Facilities]," *Transfusion Clinique et Biologique: Journal de la Societe Francaise de Transfusion Sanguine*, Vol. 16. No. 1, pp. 21–29. As of October 17, 2016:
http://www.sciencedirect.com/science/article/pii/S1246782009000093

Radnofsky, Louise, "Bloodless Pressure: More Surgery Without Transfusions," *Wall Street Journal*, April 8, 2013. As of October 18, 2016:
http://www.wsj.com/articles/SB10001424127887323494504578340962879110432

Riley, W., M. Schwei, and J. McCullough, "The United States' Potential Blood Donor Pool: Estimating the Prevalence of Donor-Exclusion Factors on the Pool of Potential Donors," *Transfusion*, Vol. 47, No. 7, 2007, pp. 1180–1188.

Russo, C. Allison, and Anne Elixhauser, "Hospitalizations in the Elderly Population, 2003," Statistical Brief No. 6, Agency for Healthcare Research and Quality, May 2006. As of October 10, 2016:
http://www.hcup-us.ahrq.gov/reports/statbriefs/sb6.jsp

Ryan, G. W., and H. R. Bernard, "Techniques to Identify Themes," *Field Methods*, Vol. 15, No. 1, 2003, pp. 85–109.

Schmidt, P. J., "Blood and Disaster—Supply and Demand," *New England Journal of Medicine*, Vol. 346, No. 8, 2002, p. 617.

Schultz, Carl H., Kristi L. Koenig, and Eric K. Noji, "A Medical Disaster Response to Reduce Immediate Mortality After an Earthquake," *New England Journal of Medicine*, Vol. 334, No. 7, 1996, pp. 438–444.

Shander, Aryeh, Axel Hofmann, Hans Gombotz, Oliver M. Theusinger, and Donat R. Spahn, "Estimating the Cost of Blood: Past, Present, and Future Directions," *Best Practice and Research Clinical Anaesthesiology*, Vol. 21, No. 2, June 2007, pp. 271–289. As of October 18, 2016:
https://www.ncbi.nlm.nih.gov/pubmed/17650777

Shander, Aryeh, Axel Hofmann, Sherri Ozawa, Oliver M. Theusinger, Hans Gombotz, and Donat R. Spahn, "Activity-Based Costs of Blood Transfusions in Surgical Patients at Four Hospitals," *Transfusion*, Vol. 50, No. 4, 2010, pp. 753–765. As of November 2, 2016:
https://www.ncbi.nlm.nih.gov/pubmed/20003061

Simonetti, Arianna, Richard A. Forshee, Steven A. Anderson, and Mark Walderhaug, "A Stock-And-Flow Simulation Model of the U.S. Blood Supply," *Transfusion*, Vol. 54, No. 3, Part 2, 2014, pp. 828–838.

Smith, Tammie, "A Transfusion of Vision," *Richmond Times Dispatch*, October 29, 2012.

Snyder, Edward, Susan L. Stramer, and Richard Benjamin, "The Safety of the Blood Supply—Time to Raise the Bar," *New England Journal of Medicine*, Vol. 372, No. 20, May 14, 2015, pp. 1882–1885.

Sobrino, Justin, and Shahid Shafi, "Timing and Causes of Death After Injuries," *Proceedings (Baylor University Medical Center)*, Vol. 26, No. 2, 2013, p. 120.

Spahn, D. R., and L. T. Goodnough, "Alternatives to Blood Transfusion," *Lancet*, Vol. 381, No. 9880, May 25, 2013, pp. 1855–1865.

Stanger, S. H., N. Yates, R. Wilding, and S. Cotton, "Blood Inventory Management: Hospital Best Practice," *Transfusion Medicine Reviews,* Vol. 26, No. 2, April, 2012, pp. 153–163.

Starr, Douglas, "Bad Blood: The 9/11 Blood-Donation Disaster," *The New Republic*, 2002, pp. 13–16.

Stauffer, Heather, "Blood Donors Always Needed; Health Care Local Centers See Drop in Donations Mitigating Factor What They're Trying," *LNP*, December 11, 2015.

Stramer, Susan L., F. Blaine Hollinger, Louis M. Katz, Steven Kleinman, Peyton S. Metzel, Kay R. Gregory, and Roger Y. Dodd, "Emerging Infectious Disease Agents and Their Potential Threat to Transfusion Safety," *Transfusion*, Vol. 49, No. s2, 2009, pp. 1S–29S.

Strochlic, Nina, "Boston Marathon Explosions: The Heroes Who Responded to the Blasts," *The Daily Beast*, April 16, 2013. As of October 18, 2016:
http://www.thedailybeast.com/articles/2013/04/16/
boston-marathon-explosions-the-heroes-who-responded-to-the-blasts.html

TBNweekly.com, "OneBlood Considers Blood Bank Merger," July 30, 2014. As of May 5, 2016:
http://www.tbnweekly.com/content_articles/073014_hth-02.txt

TerumoBCT, "CaridianBCT Announces New Era of Automation and Informatics in the Blood Banking Industry," in Atreus 3C Whole Blood Processing system displayed at German Society for Transfusion Medicine (DGTI), Booth 308, Lakewood, Colo., September 12, 2008. As of October 18, 2016:
https://www.terumobct.com/location/north-america/about-terumobct/press-room/
Pages/12SEPT,2008-CaridianBCTAnnouncesNewEraofAutomationandInformaticsintheBloodBank
ingIndustry.aspx

———, "CaridianBCT's OrbiSac System Performs One Millionth Run: Major Milestone in Automation of Whole Blood Processing to Streamline Blood Center Efficiencies," Lakewood, Colo., press release, June 15, 2010. As of October 18, 2016:
https://www.terumobct.com/location/north-america/about-terumobct/press-room/Pages/
15JUN-CaridianBCTOrbiSacSystemPerformsOneMillionthRun.aspx

Toland, Bill, "To Cut Costs, More Blood Banks Merge; Officials Cite Need for New Model," *Pittsburgh Post-Gazette*, July 31, 2014.

Toner, R. W., L. Pizzi, B. Leas, S. K. Ballas, A. Quigley, and N. I. Goldfarb, "Costs to Hospitals of Acquiring and Processing Blood in the U.S.: A Survey of Hospital-Based Blood Banks and Transfusion Services," *Applied Health Economics and Health Policy,* Vol. 9, No. 1, 2011, pp. 29–37. As of October 18, 2016:
http://rd.springer.com/article/10.2165/11530740-000000000-00000

Torio, Celeste, and Brian Moore, "National Inpatient Hospital Costs: The Most Expensive Conditions by Payer, 2013," Statistical Brief No. 204, Agency for Healthcare Research and Quality, May 2016. As of October 18, 2016:
https://www.hcup-us.ahrq.gov/reports/statbriefs/sb204-Most-Expensive-Hospital-Conditions.jsp

Trigaux, Robert, "Three-Way Blood Bank Merger in Florida Yields a Behemoth," *Tampa Bay Times*, January 21, 2012a. As of May 5, 2016:
http://www.tampabay.com/news/business/
three-way-blood-bank-merger-in-florida-yields-a-behemoth/1211608

———, "After This Mega-Deal, Call Them Big Blood," *Tampa Bay Times*, January 22, 2012b.

U.S. Department of Defense, *Department of Defense Instruction 6480.04: Armed Services Blood Program Operational Procedures*, Washington, D.C., 2013. As of November 4, 2015:
http://www.dtic.mil/whs/directives/corres/pdf/648004p.pdf

U.S. Department of Health and Human Services, *The 2005 National Blood Collection and Utilization Survey Report,* Washington, D.C.: U.S. Department of Health and Human Services, Office of the Assistant Secretary of Health, 2005.

———, *The 2007 National Blood Collection and Utilization Survey Report,* Washington, D.C.: U.S. Deparment of Health and Human Services, Office of the Assistant Secretary of Health, 2007.

———, *Biovigilance in the United States: Efforts to Bridge a Critical Gap in Patient Safety and Donor Health,* Washington, D.C.: U.S. Department of Health and Human Services, 2009. As of October 18, 2016:
https://wayback.archive-it.org/3922/20140403203201/http://www.hhs.gov/ash/bloodsafety/biovigilance/ash_to_acbsa_oct_2009.pdf

———, *The 2009 National Blood Collection and Utilization Survey Report,* Washington, D.C.: U.S. Deparment of Health and Human Services, Office of the Assistant Secretary of Health, 2011a. As of October 24, 2016:
https://wayback.archive-it.org/3919/20140402175927/https:/www.hhs.gov/ash/bloodsafety/2009nbcus.pdf

———, *The 2011 National Blood Collection and Utilization Survey Report,* Washington, D.C.: U.S. Department of Health and Human Services, Office of the Assistant Secretary of Health, 2011b. As of October 24, 2016:
http://www.hhs.gov/ash/bloodsafety/2011-nbcus.pdf

———, *The 2013 National Blood Collection and Utilization Survey Report,* Washington, D.C.: U.S. Department of Health and Human Services, Office of Assistant Secretary of Health, 2013.

———, "Permanent Discontinuance or Interruption in Manufacturing of Certain Drug or Biological Products," *Federal Register,* Vol. 80, No. 130, July 8, 2015. As of October 18, 2016:
http://www.gpo.gov/fdsys/pkg/FR-2015-07-08/pdf/2015-16659.pdf

———, "Medicaid Program; Final FY 2013 and Preliminary FY 2015 Disproportionate Share Hospital Allotments, and Final FY 2013 and Preliminary FY 2015 Institutions for Mental Diseases Disproportionate Share Hospital Limits," *Federal Register,* Vol. 81, No. 21, February 2016. As of October 18, 2016:
https://www.gpo.gov/fdsys/pkg/FR-2016-02-02/pdf/2016-01836.pdf

———, Office of the HIV/AIDS and Infectious Disease Policy, "Recommendations of the 47th Meeting of the ACBTSA, November 9–10, 2015," November 2015. As of October 18, 2016:
http://www.hhs.gov/ash/bloodsafety/advisorycommittee/recommendations/nov2015-recommendations.html.html

U.S. Department of Health and Human Services Press Office, "HHS Ships Blood Products to Puerto Rico in Response to Zika Outbreak," press release, March 7, 2016. As of October 24, 2016:
http://www.hhs.gov/about/news/2016/03/07/hhs-ships-blood-products-puerto-rico-response-zika-outbreak.html

U.S. Department of Veterans Affairs, "VBECS Blood Bank Software," Washington, D.C., 2007. As of December 14, 2015:
http://www.va.gov/vhapublications/ViewPublication.asp?pub_ID=1617

———, *Audit of Veterans Health Administration Blood Bank Modernization Project,* Washington, D.C., Office of Inspector General, No. 06-03424-70, February 8, 2008. As of December 14, 2015:
http://www.va.gov/oig/52/reports/2008/VAOIG-06-03424-70.pdf

U.S. Food and Drug Administration, Establishment Registration and Product Listing for Manufactures of Human Blood and Blood Products, Title 21, Code of Federal Regulations, Part 607, undated-a. As of October 16, 2016:
http://www.accessdata.fda.gov/scripts/cdrh/cfdocs/cfcfr/CFRSearch.cfm?CFRPart=607

————, Food and Drugs, Code of Federal Regulations, Title 21, Part 640.3, Suitability of Donor, 1999. As of October 16, 2016:
https://www.gpo.gov/fdsys/search/pagedetails.action?browsePath=Title+21%2FChapter%2FSub chapter+F%2FPart+640%2FSubpart+A%2FSection+640.3&granuleId=CFR-1999-title21-vol7-sec640-3&packageId=CFR-1999-title21-vol7&collapse=true&fromBrowse=true&collectionCode=CFR

————, "Guidance for Industry: Nucleic Acid Testing (NAT) for Human Immunodeficiency Virus Type 1 (HIV-1) and Hepatitis C Virus (HCV): Testing, Product Disposition, and Donor Deferral and Reentry," Silver Spring, Md., May 2010. As of January 13, 2016:
http://www.fda.gov/downloads/BiologicsBloodVaccines/
GuidanceComplianceRegulatoryInformation/Guidances/Blood/UCM210270.pdf

————, "VistA Blood Establishment Computer Software (VBECS), 2.0.0," November 26, 2014a. As of December 14, 2015:
http://www.fda.gov/BiologicsBloodVaccines/BloodBloodProducts/ApprovedProducts/
SubstantiallyEquivalent510kDeviceInformation/ucm424988.htm

————, "Changes to an Approved Application: Biological Products: Human Blood and Blood Components Intended for Transfusion or for Further Manufacture; Guidance for Industry," Center for Biologics Evaluation and Research, December 2014b. As of October 10, 2016:
http://www.fda.gov/downloads/BiologicsBloodVaccines/
GuidanceComplianceRegulatoryInformation/Guidances/Blood/UCM354668.pdf

————, "Requirements for Blood and Blood Components Intended for Transfusion or for Further Manufacturing Use," *Federal Register*, Vol. 80, No. 99, May 22, 2015a. As of October 10, 2016:
https://www.gpo.gov/fdsys/pkg/FR-2015-05-22/pdf/2015-12228.pdf

————, "Recommendations for Assessment of Blood Donor Suitability, Donor Deferral and Blood Product Management in Response to Ebola Virus: Draft Guidance for Industry," Center for Biologics Evaluation and Research, December 2015b. As of October 10, 2016:
http://www.fda.gov/downloads/BiologicsBloodVaccines/
GuidanceComplianceRegulatoryInformation/Guidances/Blood/UCM475072.pdf

————, "Blood Establishment Registration Database," updated as of January 8, 2016a. As of October 10, 2016:
https://www.accessdata.fda.gov/scripts/cber/CFAppsPub/Index.cfm

————, "Implementation of Acceptable Full-Length and Abbreviated Donor History Questionnaires and Accompanying Materials for Use in Screening Donors of Source Plasma: Guidance for Industry," July 2016b. As of October 25, 2016:
http://www.fda.gov/downloads/BiologicsBloodVaccines/BloodBloodProducts/ApprovedProducts/
LicensedProductsBLAs/BloodDonorScreening/UCM341088.pdf

————, "Urgent Recall Extension for Leukotrap RC System with RC2D Filter," press release, June 20, 2016c. As of November 4, 2016:
http://www.fda.gov/BiologicsBloodVaccines/SafetyAvailability/Recalls/ucm507900.htm

U.S. General Accounting Office, "Blood Supply Generally Adequate Despite New Donor Restrictions," GAO-02-754. Washington, D.C., July 22, 2002. As of October 10, 2016:
http://www.gao.gov/assets/240/235235.html

U.S. Geological Survey, "2008 Bay Area Earthquake Probabilities," last revised June 30, 2016. As of October 18, 2016:
http://earthquake.usgs.gov/regional/nca/ucerf/

U.S. National Library of Medicine, "Blood Donation Before Surgery," 2015. As of December 2, 2015:
https://www.nlm.nih.gov/medlineplus/ency/patientinstructions/000367.htm

Varricchio, Lilian, and Anna Rita Migliaccio, "The Role of Glucocorticoid Receptor (GR) Polymorphisms in Human Erythropoiesis," *American Journal of Blood Research*, Vol. 4, No. 2, 2014, p. 53. As of October 18, 2016:
http://www.ncbi.nlm.nih.gov/pmc/articles/PMC4348794/

Vaslef, Steven N., Nancy W. Knudsen, Patrick J. Neligan, and Mark W. Sebastian, "Massive Transfusion Exceeding 50 Units of Blood Products in Trauma Patients," *Journal of Trauma and Acute Care Surgery*, Vol. 53, No. 2, 2002, pp. 291–296.

Wall, J. K., "Outlook Gloomy for Medical Device Investments," *Indianapolis Business Journal*, November 2012.

Wennberg, J. E., "Appendix on the Geography of Health Care in the United States," *Dartmouth Atlas of Health Care in the United States*, 1990, pp. 289–296.

WHO—*See* World Health Organization.

Williamson, Lorna M., and Dana V. Devine, "Challenges in the Management of the Blood Supply," *Lancet,* Vol. 381, No. 9880, May 25, 2013, pp. 1866–1875. As of October 18, 2016:
http://ac.els-cdn.com/S0140673613606315/1-s2.0-S0140673613606315-main.pdf?_tid=9361aea6-833c-11e5-9211-00000aab0f6c&acdnat=1446673369_3f9dd4e96aed0c52a4f275b7d5c76ce0

Wondra, Linda, "Jonathan M. Wainwright Memorial VA Medical Center: Be Special—Donate Blood," Walla Walla Veterans Affairs Public Affairs Office, June 4, 2013. As of October 24, 2016:
http://www.wallawalla.va.gov/features/Blood_Drive_061313.asp

Wood, Erica M., Lisa J. Stevenson, Simon A. Brown, and Christopher J. Hogan, "The Australian Hemovigilance System," *Hemovigilance: A Tool for Improving Transfusion Safety,* Wiley-Blackwell, 2012, pp. 209–219. As of October 18, 2016:
http://dx.doi.org/10.1002/9781118338179.ch18

World Bank, "World Bank Open Data," undated. As of October 18, 2016:
http://data.worldbank.org/

World Health Organization, "Global Database on Blood Safety," undated-a. As of October 18, 2016:
http://www.who.int/bloodsafety/global_database/en/

———, "Global Harmonization Task Force (GHTF)," undated-b. As of October 18, 2016:
http://www.who.int/medical_devices/collaborations/force/en/

———, "Blood Safety: Key Global Fact and Figures in 2011," Fact Sheet 279, June 2011a. As of October 18, 2016:
http://www.who.int/worldblooddonorday/media/who_blood_safety_factsheet_2011.pdf

———, *Global Database on Blood Safety: Summary Report 2011*, Geneva, Switzerland, 2011b. As of December 2, 2015:
http://www.who.int/bloodsafety/global_database/GDBS_Summary_Report_2011.pdf?ua=1

———, Regional Office for South-East Asia, "Pandemic H1N1 2009," New Delhi, India, 2009. As of October 18, 2016:
http://www.who.int/iris/handle/10665/205605

Zadvydas, Thomas, "Sense of the Markets: Clarity Drives Medtech Deals," *Daily Deal/The Deal*, May 10, 2010.

Zimrin, Ann B., and John R. Hess, "Planning for Pandemic Influenza: Effect of a Pandemic on the Supply and Demand for Blood Products in the United States," *Transfusion*, Vol. 47, No. 6, 2007, pp. 1071–1079.

Zou, Shimian, "Potential Impact of Pandemic Influenza on Blood Safety and Availability," *Transfusion Medicine Reviews*, Vol. 20, No. 3, July 2006, pp. 181–189. As of October 19, 2016: http://www.sciencedirect.com/science/article/pii/S0887796306000113

Zou, Shimian, Fatemeh Musavi, Edward P. Notari, Chyang T. Fang, and ARCNET Research Group, "Changing Age Distribution of the Blood Donor Population in the United States," *Transfusion*, Vol. 48, No. 2, 2008, pp. 251–257. As of October 18, 2016: https://www.ncbi.nlm.nih.gov/pubmed/18005327